Raymond William Firth

HUMAN TYPES

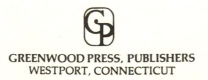

GREENWOOD PRESS, PUBLISHERS
WESTPORT, CONNECTICUT

Library of Congress Cataloging in Publication Data

Firth, Raymond William, 1901–
  Human types.

    Reprint. Originally published: London : Sphere
Books, 1975.
    Bibliography: p.
    Includes index.
    1. Ethnology.   I. Title.
GN315.F48 1983   306   83-13026
ISBN 0-313-24176-7

ABACUS revised edition published in 1975 by Sphere Books Ltd.
Sphere Books edition first published in 1970

First published in Great Britain by Thomas Nelson and Sons Ltd 1938

Revised and enlarged edition 1956
Copyright © Raymond Firth 1938, 1970 and 1975
All photographs © by Raymond Firth

Reprinted with the permission of Thomas Nelson & Sons Ltd

Reprinted from an original copy in the collection of the author

Reprinted in 1983 by Greenwood Press
A division of Congressional Information Service, Inc.
88 Post Road West, Westport, Connecticut 06881

Printed in the United States of America

10 9 8 7 6 5 4 3 2 1

Contents

5

List of Illustrations

7

Acknowledgments

For help in preparation of the original text of this work I am indebted to Dr G. M. Morant, Professor V. G. J. Sheddick, and especially to Professor W. E. H. Stanner. For advice on a later revised edition I owe thanks to Professor Maurice Freedman, Professor I. Schapera and Professor M. N. Srinivas. The present edition, like the others which preceded it, has benefited much from the critical scrutiny and encouragement of my wife, Rosemary Firth, as from her practical experience of teaching in the fields covered in this book.

Raymond Firth, 1974

Introduction

I have been pleased to find that the publishers wish to reissue this book, since it was originally written so long ago. But the fact that it has been translated into nine European and Oriental languages, apart from a continuing demand for it in Britain, seems to indicate that it has filled a need for a relatively clear, simple account of what social anthropology is about, and its meaning in the modern world.

Let me first make a disclaimer and say what this book does *not* aim to do. In the nearly forty years since this book first appeared, social anthropology has become vastly more sophisticated and more complex. The development of economic anthropology and of political anthropology was to be expected. This has given more refined exploration of the theory of decision-making, transactions and exchange, and of the processes and structures involved in the attainment, retention and manipulation of power. There have also been much more elaborate descriptive and analytical studies of religion, as well as of such special features as witchcraft. But increasingly claims have been pressed for more precise methods of analysis, both qualitative and quantitative. In particular, much greater attention has been paid not only to the ways in which people act in social situations but also to what they think and believe. So social anthropology has had to take account of ethnoscience, of cognitive anthropology, of symbolic anthropology, of socio-linguistics, of formal ethnography. Overriding them all in calling for attention as a method of study by dialectical opposition, and as a theory of the operations of the human mind, has been the idea of structuralism. Assertive, too, in demanding a thorough-going revision of our way of thinking about anthropological data as an intellectualised Marxist approach.

This book is not about these theories and methods; it is about people in society – their institutions, their patterns of thinking and behaving – based mainly upon a great range of field studies. Naturally, I had a framework of theoretical ideas in mind when writing it, and some of this comes through in my arrangement of topics, my

11

selection of examples and my interpretation of the data. Some of the changes in my thinking as time has passed have been reflected too in modifications of the original edition. But the main message of the book is the same. It is that with the diversity of types of human society, a special effort of understanding is needed to accompany judgment. To enter the way of understanding, a systematic frame-work of study is necessary, and such a framework is provided by social anthropology, which is a comparative study of custom. An important part of the message is that social anthropology is not just about exotic peoples. It applies to all human societies – though studies in highly differentiated western or oriental societies may be especially hard to make. Social anthropology is about 'us' as well as about 'them'. And ways of behaving in western societies can be just as odd or irrational to an outside observer as those in the most exotic society from Africa or the South Seas. In this sense the evidence on which my generalisations have been based is still valid.

A primary theme of this book is description and interpretation of variation in social institutions of men in different conditions, as it were on a single time-plane. But as the last chapter especially indi-cates, a great deal of social anthropology is concerned with change in institutions over time.

This is illustrated very well by modifications that have taken place in behaviour and belief in regard to some of the examples given in the introductory pages of the first chapter of this book (see pp. 21–2). In Europe and North America the wearing of trousers by women is no longer thought quaint; sex relations between young people before marriage are if not expected at least tolerated, even by the parents of the young man and woman concerned; and the strict Roman Catholic Christian is no longer debarred from eating meat on Fridays. It is interesting to note that the precipitant cause of the change has been of a different order in each case. In Britain, certainly, realisation of the practical value of wearing trousers was borne in upon women especially during the war. With the enormously in-creased entry of women into industry and allied employment the notion that a woman who wore trousers was 'mannish' receded, and the description of a dominating wife as one 'who wore the trousers' in the household ceased to have meaning. With the coming of 'jeans' as a nether garment (a good old-fashioned term) for young people of both sexes the important diacritical index of skirt *v.* trousers largely lapsed. So a superficial change in an item of clothing has been associated with a deeper change in the concept of recognition of norms of sex difference.

The growth of toleration of pre-marital freedom has been associated indirectly with material changes. The greater availability of motor transport, especially motor cycles, has enabled young people to evade the chaperonage of their elders more easily. More important, probably, has been the availability of reasonably reliable contraceptives at a low price. But its correlates of great importance have been changes in the authority roles and ideas in the family; the overt emergence of more individual control of earnings by young people; a lessening of the moral and religious sanctions for conduct, including sexual conduct; and a pervasive greater willingness, influenced ultimately to a significant extent by the views of Freud, to discuss issues of sexual association in more rational, less emotional terms.

The change from prohibiting Catholics from eating meat on Fridays to permitting them was finally triggered off by the rescinding of a religious edict by papal authority. But it came as one result of a long process of attempts to modernise the Church, and was associated more or less directly with such phenomena as vernacularisation of the Mass, struggles of some priests to marry and enjoy normal family life, and even modes of combination of Christian teaching about social justice with Marxist ideology.

Of much greater general social importance, if much less radical, have been changes in attitudes towards problems of race relations. Notably in the southern United States of America, legal and some social restrictions which formally operated to hamper the development and co-operation of Afro-Americans have ceased to apply, the majority of such racist barriers having been successfully destroyed over the last decade by the Civil Rights Movement. In Britain the change has taken another form. With a massive immigration of West Indians, and later of Asians, after the war, and an increasing population of locally born 'coloured' people, the issues of racial awareness and racial friction have come to the surface more openly, and have attracted official attention, as well as the critical study of social scientists. The creation of a Race Relations Board and related measures, while of limited effectiveness and subject to much criti-

13

cism, have been explicit attempts to give public and legal validity to concepts of racial equality as an official policy and a social commitment.

A most marked institutional change all over the world has been the abandonment of colonialism as an overt and approved system of political dominance over other people's developments. Political independence has come to nearly all Asian and African peoples who were formerly under colonial rule and most of the larger Oceanic societies have also become autonomous. Unacknowledged political suzerainty still exists in some cases of 'autonomous republics' which are satellite states or otherwise subordinate members of a federation led by a major power, and 'trusteeship' of some territories is largely a perpetuation of colonialist control. Economic dominance in what it is now fashionable to call neo-colonialism, but which has long existed in other forms, still continues in many fields. But given such restrictions on their freedom, most of the new states have seen radical changes in their social structure as modern political parties emerge, as an indigenous bureaucracy takes over the administration, as local élite and middle-class groups expand, and as problems of technical and economic development, with accompanying urbanisation and related issues take on a more local colour.

And yet beneath all such changes there is still much continuity. Look at the examples of change I have just cited.

When western women took to wearing trousers for many activities they did not sacrifice their femininity in other ways. Despite some public display of 'topless' garments, a western woman in a bathing dress on a beach still normally has her breasts covered, while a man is bare to the waist. Adoption of the male stereotype goes only a limited way. And in adopting this stereotype, women have not been abdicating from their separate rôle, but emphasising it, proclaiming their right to equality with men. Note too that except in special cases – as with Scotsmen, Greek Evzones, priests and friars, some (mainly comic) stage rôles, and the ambiguous 'drag' behaviour of some homosexuals – skirts are regarded as definitely improper wear for men, whereas they are still the most approved garment for women. In the sphere of sex relations too there is still much continuity in behaviour and moral attitudes. Despite a much more tolerant view of pre-marital living together by young men and women,

14

western society has still maintained a strong belief in the propriety if not the sanctity of the monogamous marriage tie. Nowhere in the western world is any tolerance shown towards a man contracting a marriage tie with more than one wife, or a woman with more than one husband. An extra-marital liaison may be winked at, but breach of the norm of monogamy is both a moral lapse and a criminal offence in the eyes of the law. For divorce too there is often still deep-rooted social disapproval, though the legal impediments have been much eased. It is often regarded as 'bad manners' to mention a divorced spouse of husband or wife to the present spouse; the idea of conjoining two living spouses to the same mate in the same social context is embarrassing to many people. So the much-vaunted changes in sexual mores have swirled around the idea of marriage, but have not moved the rock of monogamy.

In Catholic beliefs about the eating of flesh too there is one fundamental continuity. Despite the major change in practice about permitting the eating of flesh in an ordinary meal on Fridays, that is, an alteration in the meaning of actual flesh as a ritual symbol of indulgence, the basic significance of the eating of mystical flesh in Holy Communion remains as before. The communicant continues to believe that in partaking of the Host he is partaking of the body of the Saviour, the Lord's Anointed, but that which he perceives with his senses is not flesh but bread, which serves as a veil for the mystical substance ingested. Here in the heart of western civilisation is a type of belief of a non-rational order, involving ideas of transformation which do not conform to ordinary physical laws – a belief which has persisted over many centuries, and which has many analogues in the belief systems of other societies.

In race relations, even though great changes have occurred in the overt, formal, legal fields, prejudice and discrimination still persist widely, with skin colour and other physical characters as critical indices for social attitudes. In the United States of America, though earnest efforts have been made by many responsible citizens, both black and white, to promote racial equality, deep-rooted suspicions still exist, and conflicts over schooling, job opportunities, 'Black Studies' in universities, and the activities of Black Muslim and 'Black Power' groups exemplify this. The problems do not end there: the struggles of Puerto Ricans, of 'Chicanos' and others of Spanish-

15

American origin, and of various oriental groups in the United States to attain what they regard as proper treatment all have a component of racial antagonism to meet. Elsewhere throughout the world, the problems of ethnic minorities such as the Maori of New Zealand, the Indians of Canada and the United States, the Australian aborigines, the Nagas of Assam, the Miao and other non-Han groups of China, all involve elements of what may be called race relations. In Britain, as we are now well aware, the spate of books and articles in what has been termed almost a race relations industry indicates the sensitivity of the situation and the persistence of overt as well as underlying attitudes of prejudice.

Developments in the new states which have emerged to political autonomy after the war have been rapid and spectacular. Yet even here, elements of the former structure of the society often persist. In the effort to shape a new social identity which will be different from that recognised under the former controlling power, traditional institutions are often prized and utilised – sometimes also revived. Factional struggles for power often follow traditional tribal, clan or local groupings. And in carrying on business or conducting private affairs people are still apt to use the traditional patterns and ideas of social and ritual behaviour to which they attach great value, as being right and proper.

It has recently been said by some critics that social anthropologists have pursued their study in a colonialist framework, and that if these anthropologists have not actively supported colonialist régimes they have at least tolerated them, and not protested against racist attitudes and other aspects of domination and exploitation. Like many other social anthropologists, I have worked for some time in colonial territories, and have therefore of necessity conformed to the major structural requirements of the situation. But while I made no effort to write this book as propaganda or social protest, I have not concealed my humanist views on such issues. Any reader who follows my argument will see clearly how right from the beginning of the book I have tried to expose the weaknesses of colonialist and allied types of exploitation; to criticise racist thinking; to interpret the institutions of people in alien societies; to suggest that however small be their community, every such people is entitled to consideration; and to show how western ways of behaving and thinking which we regard as so

16

natural, so axiomatic, can be founded on nothing more elevated than self-interest or on some non-rational assumptions.

Enough changes have been taking place superficially in the social and economic life of almost any people over the last few decades to make any purely ethnographic account, from a descriptive point of view, out-of-date in a few years. But as I have indicated, much of the material I have given in this book is illustrative of general principles of social thought and action. So while I have added brief sections in some parts of the book to supplement this Introduction, and have modified some of the phrasing in other parts, I have left the body of the text in its original form as historical examples of variation in basic attitudes and institutions – as pertinent illustrations of 'human types'.

One principal modification I have made in phrasing is a reflection of a change of great interest, in the general labels used to describe the primary materials of our study – the words used for the broad category of alien or exotic societies and cultures which have formed much of the research field of the anthropologist.

The terms 'primitive', 'savage' and 'native', which were widely current as recently as thirty years or so ago as contrast to 'civilised', i.e. primarily western and Asian developed cultures, have become no longer appropriate. They are not only old-fashioned, they are also felt to be derogatory. Anthropologists have often explained that by 'primitive' they meant simply a reference to lack of technical development, without implication for social, moral or religious development. 'Primitive' kinship systems, for instance, are often very complex, far more so than western systems; and 'primitive' religious ideas are often of considerable sophistication and depth of meaning. But the meaning of the term often remained confused for non-anthropologists. And technical development has been so rapid and extensive, whether on remote Pacific islands or in the heart of Africa, that 'primitive', even in this sense, is not correct. So the term is now best abandoned. The word 'savage', of earlier currency than 'primitive' is in much the same case. Formerly equated with tropical nudity or grass skirts, with weapons of clubs or spears, savagery had as its hallmark violence as a socially recognised form of social control or reaction to an external threat. But even leaving aside the traumatic experiences of the last war, one can find so many evidences of terror-

17

ism, torture and other forms of political violence in western countries, that it is meaningless or hypocritical to apply the term to the incidental behaviour of relatively peaceful Africans or South Sea islanders. So for general use in application to types of society or culture, the term 'savage' has been dropped by anthropologists. (Its use by the distinguished French anthropologist Claude Lévi-Strauss is a special case. The original title of his book *La Pensée Sauvage*, translated into English as *The Savage Mind*, embodies a punning reference to the wild violet [pansy], illustrated on the dust jacket. It deals not with the minds of 'savages' as men different from ourselves, but with those basic, wild, 'savage' elements of thought in all men which, largely unperceived, lie at the root of much of our classification of phenomena in the world around us. 'Wild Thought' in the sense of uncontrolled basic thought process is the equivalent of 'savage' here.)

'Native' is more neutral. It is still used often in English to indicate simply local origins, with connotations of local knowledge and sharing of an individual form of culture with other local people. It is equivalent in some contexts to 'traditional'. This is the sense in which anthropologists long used the term. But there is a difference between being a native of X–, and being just a 'native' of a place unspecified. As the latter it became primarily a term of differentiation, implying not only local knowledge and culture, but also the limitations of such, viewed from the standpoint of an outside observer. Hence, when used especially by colonialists abroad, 'a native' or 'the Native' became a derogatory term, even a term of social stratification. So this too has largely passed out of anthropological use.

This successive whittling away of descriptive coverage in their general terms has left anthropologists in somewhat of a quandary. For a time they attempted to solve it by using the word 'pre-literate' for most of the subjects of their study, in cultures which did not practise the art of writing. But as education has advanced, especially rapidly in recent decades in many parts of the world, the appropriateness of this term too has receded. The term 'non-western peoples', which has tended to replace it, has the advantage of a geographical rather than a cultural reference, and is therefore less liable to alteration in people's behaviour. But it is open to objection in that it lacks content; it is unsatisfactory to define a range of societies and

18

cultures by a negative. The result has been to seek descriptive terms in more positive, if more restricted local labels. In the present edition of this book I have adopted these latter conventions where possible.

The term 'Negro' has been the object of much more active and emotional interest by non-anthropologists. An ultimate derivative from Latin, its conventional meaning was originally simply 'black'. But applied to people of dark skin colour it came to be applied primarily to the inhabitants of Africa south of the Sahara, and to the descendants of Africans taken as slaves to America. As a technical word in physical anthropology, Negro has received a fairly precise definition in terms of criteria of skin colour, hair form, physique, and its application has been extended beyond the African and directly related areas. Negroid features have been recognised, for example, among Papuans, who have sometimes been classified among Oceanic Negroids. As a term for the physical classification of peoples, 'Negro' is presumably still valid. But socially, objection has been taken to it quite strongly, on account of its unhappy associations, especially in the New World. Hence in the United States, and also more widely, the term 'Black' has come into use. This has indicated an assertion of pride – for example in the expression 'Black is beautiful', or in the poem *The Black Christ* by the black poet Countee Cullen many years ago. It has also expressed a direct challenge to White assumptions of superiority and supremacy, as in the 'Black Power' movement. 'Black' is an affirmation of identity by direct, not indirect contrast, as 'Negro' would be. Use of 'Black' instead of 'Negro' then is a recognition of the right of a people to define their own identity by what they consider to be the most suitable name. (In a similar way, many of the new nations have adopted names different from those by which their territory was formerly known, names which mark their change of state, and which often have reference to the traditional circumstances of their people: e.g. Ghana instead of Gold Coast; Zambia instead of Northern Rhodesia; Sri Lanka instead of Ceylon.)

But 'Black' is primarily a term of social and political definition; it is not strictly speaking a racial term. Many people in the United States, for instance, who have had Caucasian as well as African ancestors, are quite light-skinned in colour. If they call themselves 'Black', as many are willing to do, this is to be understood as a social and political statement, largely in reaction to Whites and to a former

19

White classification of anyone with such mixed ancestry as Negro. Not all Americans who have had some African ancestors agree with this blanket use of the term 'Black'. If they wish to identify themselves by reference to their African descent, then they see a case for a more neutral term, Afro-American. This reference to country of ultimate origin of some of their ancestors is parallel to other geographical designations, such as Spanish-American, Japanese-American, German-American. In conformity with modern taste I have adopted the usages mentioned above as seems appropriate.

I have made a few other changes in the present edition. I have retained most of the photographic illustrations which appeared in the 1956 edition of the book, but have substituted several of more direct relevance to some of the topics discussed. I have also omitted the bulk of references to older literature and replaced these by a shorter list of modern publications which will allow the reader to follow the analyses in this book further on both a descriptive and a theoretical level.

With the development of a wider public interest in anthropology, and its growing use as an educational medium, alongside history and geography, outside as well as within the universities, I hope that in its present form the book may continue to serve as an aid to understanding our own and other people's social ways of thought and action.

CHAPTER ONE

Racial Traits and Mental Differences

IN greeting each other Englishmen shake hands; Frenchmen in exalted moments embrace and kiss on both cheeks; a polite Austrian salutes a lady's hand with his lips; and Polynesians press noses. Each of these different codes of manners seems reasonable to those who practise it, but to the others who do not it is looked upon with amusement or ridicule.[1]

In much of India and the Muslim world women still veil the face as well as the body; in Europe they cover the body but expose the face; in many parts of Africa and the South Seas they leave the breasts bare, and in some regions they go entirely naked. In each case no shame is felt by the people themselves, though we think veiling the face stupid, and baring the genitalia improper. When Chinese and Eskimo women wear trousers we think it quaint, yet in Europe women may wear them for sport or work because they are more practical (see Introduction).

Differences in more fundamental sex relations arouse our deep emotions. In western civilisation monogamy is the ideal form of marriage, enforced by the Law and the Church. Elsewhere polygamy is often common, but we think it disgusting and immoral, though some countries allow it by their religion, and others justify it for economic reasons or for the preservation of the health of the growing child. In Europe again the moral code upholds chastity for both sexes before marriage, though in practice it is relaxed for men, and is now less strict than formerly for women. In many Pacific and African communities pre-marital sex relations are expected of young people. They hold that in these matters experience teaches, while we feel that in this a little learning is a dangerous sin.

The religions of the world, in spite of their many common elements, show equally deep-seated differences of belief and practice. Philosophers and theologians may agree upon the fundamentals of faith, but the ordinary man clings to his taboos in the conviction that they are sensible and right. The strict Muslim may eat no pork, the strict Hindu no beef; but the strict Christian may eat both – except perhaps on Fridays. The Brahmanic bull of Hindu India swings through the bazaar and eats his fill; the European sees in him a wasteful concession to religious prejudice, and thinks how much better he would be occupied in pulling a plough or converted into steaks. The protest of the Hindu orthodox groups of northern India against the public ox-roasting proposed in 1937 to celebrate the Coronation of their Majesties in Great Britain must have seemed comic to many Englishmen. A tradition of beef-eating, plus a religion deeply imbued with symbolism of sacrifice and of communion through partaking of flesh and blood, finds it difficult to appreciate the sincerity of a faith which believes in bloodless offerings and in veneraton of a sacred animal. A cynical Hindu might say on the other hand that the only calf we venerate is a golden one.

What is the cause of these deeply rooted differences in the ways of life and thought of people? Is it racial inheritance, or environmental conditions, or cultural heritage? And what is the meaning of these differences? In the following chapters I shall examine these questions. Writing comparatively as an anthropologist, I shall pay much attention to the habits and customs of folk whose ways of life are alien to those of western civilisation. Not only are those ways often spectacular to seekers after novelty; not only is an understanding of them important to those who work in under-developed countries, but the study of them can throw light upon our own habits and ideas. But I also give examples from western society because we too have our customs for study.

It is common to attribute ways of life and thought which we do not fully understand to racial differences. First let us see how the race idea expresses itself in practice in some characteristic situations.

Many years ago I landed in a southern port of the United States of America, and wanted to sit down and wait for a ferry. Before me was a huge building of timber, neatly painted white, with a large notice: WHITE WAITING-ROOM. New to the ways of Americans I thought innocently for a moment how naïve was this stressing of the obvious; then I went round the other side and saw another notice: COLOURED WAITING-ROOM. Coming from New Zealand, where the Maori people

22

sat in the same waiting-rooms and railway carriages and ate in the same restaurants as the white people, I had honestly failed to recognise this first intimation of the 'colour bar'.

This was in 1924. And by 1938 I could still write that, 'as every traveller knows, in the south of the United States of America this attitude of social inequality may be carried even further. "Jim Crow" cars, in which Negroes must travel within the State boundaries; refusal of entry to hotels, restaurants, and places of amusement for white people; restrictive tests when the franchise allowed to every American citizen is sought; and (till recently) lynchings – all deny to the Negro the freedom of social and economic opportunity which other citizens possess. In the Union of South Africa, again, the colour bar is drawn; African labourers receive by law lower wage rates than white people; are not allowed to compete in the skilled trades; suffer the indignities of the "pass" control when they wish to travel or be abroad at night; and in part are subjected to territorial segregation. With this can be contrasted the position of the Negro in the North of the United States, where many of the restrictions to be found in the South do not operate; in Brazil; or in France, where a Negro vice-president of the Chamber of Deputies was applauded on his assumption of the chair by his white fellow-representatives'.

In 1942 I was in Washington, DC. There I met Dr Ralph Bunche, whom I had known briefly in London, and who was then a minor official in an intelligence service of the United States, long before his distinguished career in the United Nations. Bunche and I and an anthropological colleague went to dine together – at the railway station, which I was told was the only place in Washington where a Black and two Whites could eat together without challenge. On the way home I asked Ralph Bunche how he liked living in Washington. He told me: he and his family could not go to a cinema downtown; if his wife wanted to buy a dress she could do so only in the uptown quarter; there was a school round the corner from his house but he had to take his children right across Washington by car because the school was reserved for white children. I went up to Howard, the Negro University, to talk with colleagues, particularly with Franklin Frazier, so well-known for his studies of the Negro family in the United States. Hearing that I was from England, an anthropological colleague told me of an experience he had recently had with an

23

Englishman in one of Washington's main streets. The Englishman had said to my Black colleague, 'Let's go into this bar and have a drink.' My colleague replied, 'I can't go in there.' The Englishman said, 'What's the matter? Of course you can go in there!' not realising there was a colour bar. Then my colleague explained to me, very carefully, almost as if to a child, 'You see, he didn't know that I couldn't go in there, but I knew that I couldn't go in there.' Apart from a sense of shame, I felt I was in an almost surrealist situation. We had been discussing intellectual issues as colleagues, and suddenly one was in a realm of irrationality. There had been a door leading to a bar, and a man was unable to go through it – not physically, but socially, because he was black. I looked up at the Capitol, and thought – this is the federal capital of the United States of America, where all men are supposed to be free.

It took about twenty years after that – till about 1964 – before a radical change took place in the status of Afro-Americans in the southern United States, even in Washington. Now, as I have mentioned in the Introduction, most of the public legal and social disabilities of Afro-Americans have been removed, though many private norms of discrimination still remain.

But in the Union of South Africa the policy of *apartheid*, of separation of black and white and denial of rights to Africans, has intensified. As recently as July 1974, forcible steps were being taken by the Department of Bantu Administration to evict 12,000 Bapedi tribespeople from areas they had bought and occupied since 1905 and resettle them in a 'homeland' designated by the government for African residence.[2] This was but an incident in the grand plan of *apartheid*, which has involved the relocation – by force in many cases – of nearly two million Africans, and which has progressively barred sexual relations between black and white, excluded blacks from universities attended by white students, and generally limited the economic, social and political development of the Bantu peoples.

Why is there this denial of equality of rights to these Afro-Americans and African Bantu? The reasons lie deep, but we can see a few of them. One is deliberate exploitation; the white man wants a supply of 'cheap' labour.[3] Another is the fear of competition, both in the immediate economic sphere, and more remotely in a threat to social privilege and control. In part, too, there is conservatism, linked with a desire for the preservation of order; the domination of the white man over the black is one means of preventing a radical upheaval in which not merely one but all parties might suffer. Then there is the feeing of sex jealousy, seen in the attempts to prevent black men from having sex relations with white women, though the reverse may be winked at. Important also is the theory of trusteeship. This domination, established though it has been chiefly on a basis of material superiority, is thought to promote the material welfare, the higher ethical standards, and the greater intellectual and spiritual efficiency of the Black. Such peoples, whatever be their ultimate claims to self-government and individual expression, need, it is held, control and guidance through the difficult adjustment to civilisation; even though in time they may advance sufficiently along the road to be able to take their place side by side with their teachers – in partnership.

Sometimes one reason may be disguised in the form of another by the process which the psychologist calls a rationalisation. In April 1937 a meeting of European alluvial gold diggers in Tanganyika Territory passed a resolution protesting against the Government's policy of allowing Africans to take out prospecting rights in a controlled area. They said: 'The effect on a native of a sudden acquisition of £40 or £50 – to him comparative wealth – often turns his head, and as he quickly spends his money he is tempted to obtain more gold by illegal means.' They held that as a result of there being so many African prospectors, illicit gold-dealing had become rampant in the area; European diggers' gold was being stolen and their very existence was threatened. This plausible case for law and order, though probably quite honestly put forward, did, however, disguise perhaps even to the Europeans themselves their own self-interest in securing a monopoly.

These motives are not all of equal strength, nor do they influence all white men to the same degree. Not all European missionaries in Africa, for instance, visualise themselves as destined for ever to lead and control the local Christians. Some hold, the future of the Church in Africa must be self-government by native Africans.

It will have been noticed that in some of the conflicts of point of view already mentioned the white man sometimes tries to induce the African to adopt the white man's way of behaviour; sometimes he places every obstacle in the way of the African who wishes to imitate the white man. Here we have what might be called a theory of positive and negative race inequality. In the one case the African is regarded as being at the moment capable of better things, of being able to take on a superior way of life. On the other he is regarded as being unsuited to this way of life, or a danger to it if he enters it. The former point of view is found more particularly in areas where the Africans still retain much of their tribal way of life; the latter where they enter into direct competition with Europeans in more or less industrialised conditions. The possibility of getting even a partial solution of the 'Native problem' in areas such as South Africa is blocked to a large extent by the way in which these views cancel each other out and reduce to impotence efforts at reform.

Since what are commonly called 'racial differences' play such an important part in determining the relations between peoples, we must now examine more closely what this idea of race means. To most people it is fairly simple. They know that they can distinguish a European, or an American of that stock, on account of his fair skin, more or less wavy hair, thin lips, and narrow nose. A Negro will be recognised by his dark skin, woolly hair, thick lips, and broad nose, and a native of the Orient by his 'yellow' skin, black straight hair, flattened face, and the peculiar folded form of his eyelid. An American Indian or an aboriginal Australian may also be picked out with some assurance on account of their specific physical characters.

In broadest terms the anthropologist will usually agree with this; in fact, he will sometimes speak in terms of skin colour of the white races, the dark races, and the yellow races. Exact records are available relating to the skin, hair, and eye colours, the form of the hair, blood reactions, measurements of the size and proportions of the head and body, and numerous other physical traits for groups of living people in different parts of the world. On such bases, in a very broad sense, racial types have been recognised as: Caucasoid (Europe and descendants of Europeans elsewhere); Mongoloid (Asia and aboriginal America); Negroid (central and southern Africa); and Australoid (aboriginal Australia, parts of the western Pacific). But their distribution on the ground is very complex, and there are many intermediate types. Large numbers of skeletons representing extinct populations also have measurements and observations recorded for them.

26

It is found that the characters studied can be divided into two principal classes. The first class includes characters – such as skin colour or hair form – which make fairly clear distinctions between large groups of people such as Europeans in general and Negroes in general. These large groups, constituting major divisions of the one existing species of Man, may be called varieties. But even when all these characters are considered together it is not possible to make sharp divisions between the varieties, since some groups show a gradation between the more extreme forms.

It is also necessary to distinguish between the sub-groups within each particular variety; these are usually called races, though the term has been so misused that an alternative one, such as sub-variety or ethnic group, may be used. To recognise races a further set of characters is required. Of these stature and cephalic index – i.e. the maximum breadth of the head expressed as a percentage of its maximum length – have been historically most utilised. At the same time time the individual differences within such groups are considerable. Even when all the characters most suitable are taken into account, the anthropologist is often unable to ascertain with certainty the race to which a particular living person or skeleton belongs. Properly speaking, the idea of race should not be applied to individuals considered singly, but only to chosen groups of individuals.

Again, in defining a race it is agreed that the physical features regarded as significant must be capable of being transmitted to the descendants of the people so classified. To take the simplest case, an Austrian skier who had been burnt almost black by the sun is not therefore classified with the dark races; his sunburn will make no difference to the colour of any children he may afterwards have.

The value of head form as an index of race was called in question historically when Franz Boas, an American anthropologist, seemed to have proved that the shapes of the heads of children of immigrants born in the United States differed appreciably from the head-shapes of their European parents, presumably owing to change in environment and social conditions. When the material was re-examined, however, it was found that the differences between the two generations were not large enough to warrant the inferences drawn from them.

It is not possible as yet to answer fully the question as to how this

27

transmission of physical features takes place from one generation to another, or how exact it is. One difficulty in studying the subject is that human beings cannot be bred for experimental purposes as fruit-flies or mice have been; another is that the period between infancy and reproductive age is so long. But our studies so far, linked with those of the geneticists, show that what we call racial differences in human beings are transmitted in the form of genes, sub-microscopic factors appearing in pairs in the germ-cell, one factor in the pair being derived from each parent. It would seem that any single physical character which we take as an index of race – such as the form of the hair or the shape of the nose – is not transmitted by a single gene in each case, but by a combination of a considerable number of genes, which makes the problem more complicated to unravel. (Blood groups, however, are known to be inherited according to simple Mendelian rules.) Moreover, it is probable that genes for different types of characters are inherited separately; a particular type of hair, for instance, need not necessarily be inherited together with a particular shape of nose.

Genetical conditions which can be used with precision for racial differentiation have not yet been isolated. But the sickle cell trait seems to be a genetical condition of a racial kind. In what is known as sickle cell anaemia some red cells of the body take on an irregular curved shape which has been likened to a sickle. When there is no anaemia, but an individual's red cells can be made to assume a similar condition by special test, this is termed the sickle cell trait. Apparently the condition is found primarily in Negroes or in individuals who have some Negro ancestry. Differences in the threshold of taste, tested by a bitter substance phenyl-thio-carbamide (PTC), seem also to be transmitted and have a racial distribution.

All living human beings are classified as members of one species, *homo sapiens*, and all crosses between them seem to be fertile. Movements of population in prehistoric as well as in historic times have taken place over a wide area, and interbreeding has occurred freely. The result is that between large geographical groups of people there are no clear-cut divisions. Europeans have on the whole lighter skins, thinner lips, and narrower noses than people of the dark races, but among people with predominantly dark skins there are some whose skins are lighter than those of the darkest Europeans (though not so

28

light as those of the lightest Europeans). Again, among the people with dark skins there are some with thinner lips and narrower noses than some of the people with light skins. When stature is compared, it is found, for instance, that among the Hottentot, a short people on the whole, there are men who are taller than the shortest Europeans. Averages only, then, and not absolute differences must be used. And with each character chosen for measurement, though the averages differ, the extremes overlap. A racial or ethnic type is then a combination of averages, an abstraction, and very few individuals in a population conform precisely to the standard type. Such abstractions have to be used in order to discuss relationships between racial groups.

When it is a question of classifying all the people who live in a given country, or who share common traditions of the past, the complexity of the problem soon becomes obvious. Take two types which became a subject of bitter discussion in Europe before World War II, the Nordics and the Jews.

The Swedes are generally acknowledged to be one of the most Nordic of the European populations. Yet when Retzius and Fürst in 1897-8 measured 45,000 army conscripts of twenty-one years of age, they found that only 11 per cent of them were of the 'pure' Nordic type, with long skulls, tall stature, fair hair, and light eyes. And the maximum of 'pure' Nordics in any province was 18·3 per cent (in Dalsland). When men with the same hair and eye colour and tall stature, but with heads of medium breadth were included, the average was still only 29 per cent for the whole of Sweden, and a maximum for any province of 41·4 per cent (in Härjedalen). These conscripts would be, if anything, above the average in stature, and certainly gave a fair sample of the whole population. Thirty years later measurements of the same kind were made again in Sweden under the direction of Lundborg and Linders on 47,000 conscripts. 87 per cent of them were found to have light eyes, 8 per cent eyes of mixed shade, and 5 per cent brown eyes. But only 7 per cent had flaxen hair, and 63 per cent had light brown hair, with 25 per cent medium brown, 2 per cent brownish-black, and 3 per cent red hair. And only 30 per cent were long-headed, with 56 per cent with heads of medium ratio, and 14 per cent broad-headed. Hair and eye colour were found to be closely connected, but these together had no close connection with stature or head form. Thus the Swedes can only be described as being a 'comparatively' Nordic type, and a considerable percentage are not even that.

The Germans are even less Nordic than the Swedes, and there is a great variety of physical types among them. In the north-west particularly there are many people with long heads, tall stature, fair hair, and blue or light eyes – the Nordic type. But there and elsewhere there are many who do not fit this description. Especially in the south and east there are large numbers of people with broad skulls, brown hair, and brown eyes, and short stature. These are classed as Alpines, one of the three major racial types of Europe. Intermediate types between Nordic and Alpine are extremely common, such as people with a broad Alpine head with a long Nordic face, and they and the Alpines together outnumbered the 'pure' Nordics.

What about the Jews? Many people think that the Jews are a racial group, and that one can identify a Jew by something in his physical appearance. Investigation has shown that such identification is by no means always possible. Practically every civilised country today has its own type of Jewish people, differing considerably in physical features from the Jews in other countries. An important social distinction between Jews is whether they belong to the Ashkenazim or Sephardim, the primary distinction being one of religious practice. Outside Israel, the former are mostly in northern Europe and the United States, the latter in Italy, Spain, Portugal, and North Africa. Now, in the northern European Jews, according to Fishberg, 30 per cent were blonde in type, 50 per cent had light-coloured eyes, and on the whole they were brachycephalic, i.e. broad-headed. The southern European Jews had black hair and brown eyes, and were dolichocephalic, i.e. long-headed. In these respects Jewish populations did not show racial unity, but tended to resemble in physical features the people among whom they lived.

Outside Europe Jews have an even greater variation in physical characters. There are Berber Jews, dark Indian Jews, Chinese Jews, and a Jewish group in Ethiopia known as Falashas, all of whom resemble closely the people of these countries, perhaps through intermarriage or their own selection of certain types among themselves. The cephalic index has been a conventional index of race. Caucasian Jews have been found to have a cephalic index of 86·3, that is, they are very broad-headed. Jews of the Yemen of Arabia on the other hand have been found to have a cephalic index of 74·3, and those of the Mzab in North Africa to have a cephalic index of 72·9, that is, they are distinctly long-headed.

All this goes to show that Jewish people are not of a uniform physical type. It is true that in some countries there are certain combinations of physical features which have come to be thought of as peculiar to Jewish peoples, and in fact do characterise a certain number of Jews there. But the idea that one can always identify a Jew by these physical features is a narrow misconception which would speedily be corrected if the person who held it were to travel and try seriously to examine its accuracy. He would find, for instance, that he would be continually identifying as Jews Armenoid people from the Near East, and from the shape of their noses he would be puzzled by some dark-skinned Papuans of southern New Guinea, whom some observers have described as having a Semitic appearance.

If the Jews are not a race, then what are they? They are a cultural category based on a common religion and common traditions; and to some extent, common aspirations and ways of life. Social and economic circumstances have in addition often forced them to maintain this unity by living in segregated quarters of cities, by marrying mainly among themselves, and by getting a living in restricted fields, such as commerce. This has tended to perpetuate the idea of their being a racial group, although, in fact, they are not primarily so.

The important thing that comes out of this discussion is the clear distinction that must be drawn between a race and a nation. A race is a group of people who have certain heritable physical characters in common; a nation a group of people with certain social characters in common. Zulus, who historically have been spoken of as a nation, also form a racial group, being classified by their skin colour, shape of the head, and face. The Germans are a nation because of their common political unity, their common economic and social life, their legal system, and so on. Physically they are not a homogeneous race, since they show a great variety of physical features. So also with other countries of Europe. Terms such as 'the British race' are quite incorrect from the scientific point of view. If the user of them is challenged he will probably be found to be using the term quite vaguely, and be able to justify it only by thinking of linguistic unity in the first case, and political unity in the second. If he imagines that the inhabitants of the British Isles represent a single physical type he is quite wrong.

This example brings up the question of language. Racial classification and speech classification must not be confused. Three languages, Welsh, Gaelic, and English, are spoken in Great Britain, but the speakers of them cannot be classified simply into three physical types. The term Aryan much used in Hitlerite Germany is kept by scientists as a name for types of language only. To what original race or races the speakers of the ancient Aryan languages belonged we are not yet certain. But we are sure that the peoples of Europe who claim to be Aryan in physical type are using this term in quite a different sense from the scientific one; it must be regarded as a wish-fulfilment rather than as a statement of fact.

This leads us to a further question, that of the existence of pure human races. Even if a community of people whose ancestors are believed to have intermarried for a number of generations is examined, very considerable differences are found between the individuals composing it. All modern populations must be supposed to be very mixed from a racial point of view. The evidence of series of skeletons shows conclusively that this is not a peculiarity of modern communities, but that the situation was approximately the same two thousand years ago, and probably six thousand years ago. We have no direct evidence of any ancient populations which were markedly less variable than the existing modern ones. Hence to embark on a discussion regarding the intermixture of a number of hypothetical pure stocks is unprofitable, and there is no direct evidence whatever for the existence of 'pure' racial populations. To claim any purity of stock for a living European group is therefore ludicrous.

During the historic period, and for tens of thousands of years before, Europe has been the object of invasion from Asia and from Africa; groups have met and mingled and the result is a great mixture of types. The genes, those packets of chemical substances which are thought to determine our physical appearance, have been assembled and distributed again, combined and recombined by seventy to a hundred generations of parents since the days of Julius Caesar. The possibility, then, of modern fair-haired, blue-eyed persons having inherited those characters on both sides of the family from Julius Caesar's Gauls is extremely unlikely, and it is very probable that even

32

then some Gauls had dark hair and brown eyes. Purity of race is a concept of political propaganda, not a scientific description of human groups today.

It is necessary, then, to distinguish between the idea of race when used for the broad description of present physical differences, and when used to account for the origin of these differences in the past. We see in the world today no pure races. But it is often assumed that there were in the past such pure stocks which have intermingled to produce the existing mixed populations. It is in this inexact sense that the peoples of Europe have been classified into three major racial groups: Nordic, Alpine, and Mediterranean. In Europe, for instance, the Highland Scots, the Spaniards, the Norwegians, and the French, each of whom at times has been termed a race, all show a diversity of type at the present time. This diversity goes back a long way in history, as skeletal remains show, and even here the skeletons are not numerous enough, or sufficiently free from variation, to allow us to think we have found the original types. So also in Africa. The terms 'Hamite' and 'Negro' have been used to distinguish two great racial groups, the former to the north, the latter to the south. (Nilotic and Bantu, which broadly correspond to these in some popular contexts, are primarily linguistic terms.) But, in fact, practically every 'Negro' population shows an 'admixture' of 'Hamitic' characters, and the 'Hamites' themselves are by no means a pure race. In effect, we are explaining present variations in terms of a hypothesis of *original* stocks, the idea of which comes mainly from our separation of elements in the *present* populations. This is judging by appearances, and, in fact, ignoring the direct evidence of skeletal material. It is important to stress this point, since many people who are not biologists or anthropologists take as established results what can only be tentative ideas. When we speak of human race differences, then, we mean only a set of broad divisions, conventional and not yet established on very solid bases. We know little of race origins, and less about the possible outcome of further race mixture. We are not in the position of the biologist, who has based his divisions of plant and animal groups upon a great deal of experimental work upon the isolation of types and the effects of crossing types, and has examined closely the genetical factors responsible for the differences. This is not yet the case for our classification of human groups.

33

A word may be said about the relation of environment and physical type, which seems to be fairly clearly established on biological levels. But this relationship must not be overstressed, or the causality too precisely attributed.

The races with the heaviest skin pigment seem usually to inhabit the hot, tropical, or sub-tropical climatic zones where the actinic rays of the sun are most active. The presence of the pigment may afford them some protection from deep penetration. But this is true only of the Old World, and there are many exceptions. In the New World, at least as it was before its occupation by whites, there was no such correlation. It is thought also that there may be some relation between the size of the human nasal aperture, which differs considerably between the races, and the different degrees of humidity and temperature in different parts of the world's surface. The wide flaring nostrils of the Negro and the narrow fine nostrils of the north European represent perhaps the extremes of this feature. If it is to the advantage of the human organism to have cold air warmed by passing between heated mucous membranes before reaching the lungs, then the narrower nostrils of the north European may be said to represent a beneficial relationship between physical type and environment, just as animals which live in the snow of the Arctic have shaggy coats of hair which protect them. The presence of such adaptations in man might be predicted *a priori*. But actual *proof* that such features are environmentally determined is another matter, and for the present it appears that one cannot proceed with much validity beyond the level of correlation, as distinguished from causality.

We have seen that when the term 'race' is used scientifically, that is, with some attempt at exactness and precision, it does not give us a simple classification of peoples. But in popular discussion the word 'race' is used very broadly and often not clearly, as if it were simple in its application. Moreover, the idea of race is a powerful social force; around it cluster all kinds of prejudices, and it is made the basis of political action, which discriminates against whole groups of people. Such groups are often thought to have a peculiar mentality, to be incapable of contributing to advance in civilisation, and to have such a close relation between their psychology and their physical features that any mixture of them with other races will be a disadvantage to the latter. This has been held to be true, for instance, of Jews in Ger-

34

many, and of Negroes in the United States and South Africa.

In order to try and keep clear the distinction between these groups and the politically dominant group which sees them as a scapegoat or a threat, the exponents of these race doctrines have adopted a curious pseudo-scientific classification. All those people are classed as Jews or Negroes who have the external features of what is understood to be their general type, and in addition those people who can be found out to be descended from ancestors of this type. In practice the index for the latter is of a very limited and arbitrary kind. In Germany it ordinarily went only as far as common knowledge could trace. And when the Jewish or Negro ancestor was found, then for practical purposes the person concerned was classed as Jew or Negro. It must be emphasised that this kind of classification is a long way from a scientific one. Biologically – and 'race' to be an accurate term must be a biological one – it is impossible to put in such a crude way the immensely complicated contributions that thousands of ancestors have made to the physical and mental make-up of the person in question. No one can possibly know of a person in advance simply because he has had a Jewish or Negro grandmother what his intelligence will be like, what will be his powers of initiative and leadership, or what contributions he may make to the social life of the community in which he lives.

Where 'racial' antagonism exists it is really a social antagonism, of the same order as the clash between different national or other social groups. It is founded not on known difference of capacity and mentality between races as such, but on difference of economic and other social interests. Skin colour and other physical differences are not the real basis for the antagonism; they are merely a convenient and arbitrary symbol for it. From this point of view it could be said, as Michael Banton has done,[4] that 'race' applies to both social and physical classifications, that the two designations overlap, but that they are based on different criteria and can never be identical.

The social aspect of problems of race relations is very clear in Britain. There is a long history of British reaction to the presence of people of a different skin colour,[5] but until recently such reaction came only sporadically to public attention. In recent years the marked growth of a 'coloured' population in Britain has been accompanied by difficulties in regard to job competition, housing and school standards, felt by all parties concerned. The issues have been sharpened by what have been called racial differencs, but which are really cultural differences, since understandably most of these immigrant people wish to retain some of the styles of family life, cuisine, social and religious patterns of their former home community. The situation is very complex, since different cultural groups are involved, from the West Indies, and various parts of Asia and Africa, mainly from the Commonwealth. Each tends to meet special problems, as the Sikh men have found in trying to retain their turbans when social rules would demand uniform caps, crash helmets or other seemingly incompatible headgear. Any individual from one of such groups may suffer from or feel discriminated against by the ignorance and prejudice of some of his British fellows, but basically this is because the difference of his skin colour allows him to be taken as a symbol for a complex set of social circumstances. And in Britain, despite regrettable colour prejudice and discrimination by some people, the idea of public restrictions of the order of a 'colour bar' is abhorrent to official and most private opinion.

Let us examine the situation a little further in respect of the 'colour bar'. If it were true that dark skin, and an ancestry of dark skin, really meant some fundamental difference in outlook and capacity from white skin, then we should find the colour bar existing in all parts of the world. This is not the case. In the Union of South Africa, and formerly in the south of the United States, the colour bar has operated most stringently. But in the north of the United States, and in many parts of colonial Africa it has been much less strong. In Angola, for instance, it has been reported that a European government officer may marry an African woman and set up a household which has the respect and recognition of full social status.

The colour bar is set up in defence of vested interests. Where these interests are not thought to be threatened, where previous historical relations have tended to promote co-operation, where the dark-skinned population is small in comparison with the white population, where there is an honest attempt to apply principles of social equality and forgo the advantages of exploitation, the colour bar is lowered, or may never have been set up.

The situation varies in different communities. In New Zealand the Maori people, many of whom are now of mixed European blood, are in a position of general equality with Europeans. They number (as of 1972) about a quarter of a million in a total population of about three million. Many of them live on their own lands, in blocks, or scattered among white farmers; others are in industry, commerce, or the professions in the towns. They elect their own representatives to the New Zealand Parliament, roughly in proportion to the European representation. Their leaders are recognised for their services not only to their own people, but to the Dominion as a whole. One Maori medical man was for some time Minister of Health for the Dominion, in charge of European as well as Maori health services. In public social relations there is no discrimination: both peoples meet in hotels, restaurants, racecourses, clubs, schools, and football teams. Rather less than a century has passed since there was bitter warfare between the Europeans and some sections of the Maori people, but nowadays there is much real admiration for the Maori and their past achievements, even on the battlefield against the white people. This does not mean that all white New Zealanders have an intelligent appreciation of the needs and way of life of the Maori people; ignorance and colour prejudice exist, and admiration of the Maori is sometimes based on nothing more than respect for his sporting qualities. But, on the whole, an adjustment has been reached which allows effective co-operation.

In New Zealand the social position of the Maori is such that the offspring of mixed marriages tend on the whole to retain and stress their connection with the Maori group rather than to seek complete absorption in the European group, which is legally possible and socially has precedent.

In Hawaii, popularly called the 'melting-pot of the Pacific', there is a bewildering variety of racial intermixture. Native Hawaiians, Americans, Chinese, Japanese, Portuguese, Filipinos have all intermarried, and their offspring intermarried again, producing a wide range of physical types. There is no general theory of racial inequality or any organised public sentiment against intermarriage between members of the different groups. Friction sometimes occurs, as between the American and Japanese groups, and personal and family feeling against some marriages exists. But on the whole there is no widespread formalised objection. This situation has been attributed to a variety of historical reasons: the absence of white women at an

37

early stage of the intermixture; the marital freedom of the native Hawaiians, and their compatibility of temperament, intelligence, and physical type with those of the immigrants; the advent of the early missionaries from New England, and not from the southern United States; and the absence of a single 'dominant race'. Thus, though the groups of immigrants had each strong traditional codes of their own, which still to some extent govern the behaviour of their descendants, no real colour bar has emerged, and social contacts are free to a large extent – though the group regarded as 'native Hawaiians' and still basically of Polynesian descent, is on the whole in an economically depressed position.

These two examples show how the presence of different racial groups side by side, and their intermixture, need not be productive of clash; and that where such clash does appear, it is based upon social differences and not upon the opposition of physical types as such.

A word may be said about the position of mixed-blood peoples. It is vulgarly said: 'A half-caste has the vices of both parents and the virtues of neither.' In so far as this is true – and it may occasionally be so – it is due primarily not to the fact of being a mixed-blood, but to the social environment in which the mixed-blood grows up. Lack of proper education, no stable social position, barriers to free relationship with either his father's or his mother's people, difficulties if he wants to marry, all tend to destroy his confidence and self-esteem, and unfit him for a stable social life. The very social prejudice which condemns the instability of the mixed-blood is the cause of it.

In all these situations of colour problems and mixed-blood problems there is no sovereign remedy. Both intelligence and goodwill are necessary for the solution. The first is wanted to supply the analysis of the social forces in order that the second may work clearly.

Where the distinction between races is of social importance, and is based on a pseudo-genetic distinction, there are, of course, attempts to evade it. In the United States of America there are many people of mixed Negro descent who look like Europeans. In the past, some have taken advantage of this to pass as such. This 'passing' is a well-recognised custom and those who are too dark-skinned to attempt it themselves assist their more fortunate brethren where possible. If two members of the same family, one of whom is 'passing' with white people, and the other not, meet in public, the latter does not give the

38

former away by recognising him. A similar situation has been noted in South Africa, where it is regarded as permissible for a person of mixed blood who is 'passing' to *vensterkies*, to 'window-gaze', and ignore even his own brother in the street.[6] Such conduct is not resented; the public recognition of family ties is regarded as being of less importance at the moment than the maintenance of the position of the 'passing' member as a European. The situation may seem ridiculous to an English reader. Tragic it may be, but it is a serious and, one must say, justifiable means of evading the rigidity and stupidity of racial prejudice, and the social barriers erected upon it.

A further proof that the colour bar is in essence a culture clash, but not a racial clash as such, is seen by the revealing comments of James Weldon Johnson, a well-known Afro-American writer. Proud of his Negro ancestry, he did not accept with equanimity all the disabilities which this implied. But when travelling in the southern United States on two occasions he was saved from embarrassment and social difficulty by being mistaken for a South American. It is not colour alone that counts, but colour in a particular context. As Johnson acidly remarks: 'In such situations any kind of a Negro will do; provided he is not one who is an American citizen.'[7]

We have shown that the idea of race refers to the broad differences in physical type between peoples. A question we have now to ask is how far these differences can be seen in the composition of the mind as well. Do people in different parts of the world behave differently because their innate mental processes are unlike?

The first test that might occur to any one who wishes to find this out would be to measure the size of the brains of the different types of people. A simple way to do this is to measure the capacity of the skull by filling it with seed or some other substance which can easily be computed, or by making an endocranial cast of the inside of the skull. Differences in the proportions of the size of the brain in the gorilla, prehistoric species of man, and modern man have long been established, and Elliot Smith and others have been able to indicate those areas in each type, the expansion of which has been linked with human evolution. But so far as existing types of man are concerned, differences in brain size do not seem to be significant as an index of the relative mental capacity of races. The study of brain weights, too,

39

has not yielded any definite results. Some publicity locally was gained in East Africa for the work of Gordon and of Vint, who attempted to show that there are differences in the size, type, and rate of growth of African brains as compared with European brains. Gordon, from skull measurement, stated that the average rate of annual increase of the European brain between the ages of ten and twenty is about double that of an African brain during the same period. Vint found the average weight of the African brain to be 10·6 per cent less than the average weight of the European male adult brain. Moreover, he found a quantitative deficiency in the brain cortex of Africans of 15 per cent as compared with that of Europeans, the cells of the cortex being qualitatively deficient in size, form, and arrangement. These investigations are interesting from the anatomical point of view, and may point to valid differences. But Gordon was not content to let his conclusions rest there. He argued that if this cerebral deficiency is common in East Africa, then European methods of education of the African cannot hope to do what is intended. A number of technical objections have been raised against the work of Gordon and of Vint, but leaving these aside, one may question the value of their conclusion in the psychological field. No valid relationship between size of brain and mental capacity or intelligence has yet been proved. And still more is it impossible to proceed from brain differences to educational potentiality. In the present state of our knowledge the three levels – the anatomical, the psychological, and the cultural – have not been adequately linked.

The attempt to bring anatomy and psychology together in the study of racial differences would seem to be most fruitful in the examination, not of the mere size and weight of the brain, but of the subtlety of its structure. But here the anatomist shows the greatest caution. J. Shellshear, for instance, in a careful study of forty-four brains of Australian aborigines, pointed out that certain features of these brains do not seem to be developed to the extent that they are in European peoples; and that the most fully developed of the Australian brains would look ill-formed and under-developed as compared with, say, a fully developed Chinese brain. His conclusions broadly agreed with those of Kappers and Cunningham. But he pointed out that the crux of the problem is whether one would notice a definite difference between the most highly developed Australian brain and the least-developed normal Chinese brain. He stated clearly that from his study no solution had yet been reached on this question. He noticed also that in many works on the brain *primitiveness* (of structure) and *lowliness* (of mentality) are used as synonymous terms. But Shellshear stressed the fact that primitiveness, which means that unspecialised features have remained in the brain in process of evolution, may offer possibilities of greater evolutionary advance than the more specialised (and, therefore, 'superior') types. In commenting on Vint's work, Gordon stressed the fact that a remarkable proportion of undifferentiated cells were found in the grey matter of the African brain. He regarded this as an index of cerebral deficiency. From Shellshear's point of view it might well be a source of potential strength, allowing the African in time to rise to heights which the European with his more specialised grey matter will not reach!

Examination of the brains of different races tells us practically nothing about their mental character. Can we turn to psychology for help? A great number of tests have been worked out to measure mental traits – the acuteness of the senses; the susceptibility to fatigue; the functioning of higher mental processes like memory and the association of ideas; and even the degree of that general but elusive feature called 'intelligence'.

The wide application of difficult colour-matching tests by Woodworth led him to say that the colour sense is probably very much the same all over the world – though the classification of colour perceptions varies greatly in different cultures. So also with other senses. Little significant difference is found between civilised and primitive peoples. It is firmly believed by many people that primitive hunters in Australia or Africa are superior to white men in identification of objects or sounds at a distance. But the tests show that where this superiority exists it is due not to better faculties as such, but to attention to points which the white man overlooks – in other words, to the use of familiar clues which early training has taught to be significant. The same is true of keenness of smell. There seems to be little difference again in the sense of touch, though this has not been very fully examined. Some investigators have found that the threshold of pain appears to be higher among primitive than among civilised peoples; that is, the former stood the pressure of an instrument longer before saying they felt pain. But, as the investigators point out, this result may have been due to the fact that the white men reported the first twinge they felt, whereas the local people waited until the pressure really hurt. This points again to the difficulty of distinguishing between social and psychological factors, that is, of making sure that what is being measured is really some innate process, and not simply a way of behaving which the person has been taught to adopt.

A great deal of experimental work has been carried out in order to test the comparative intelligence of different racial groups. One difficulty here is to understand what is meant by intelligence. Many American scientists have held that there is no single mental feature which can be so called, but that there are only a number of special abilities. The view of some British scientists, notably Spearman, has been that there is a general aspect of mind which can be so called. But, broadly speaking, intelligence may be regarded as ability to learn and to use what is learned in new situations. In order to compare the intelligence of races it is necessary to study large groups of people in each. Moreover, it is important that the test shall allow each group of people to be measured in situations they are familiar with, so that they are not handicapped merely by their different ways of life.

A number of ways have been thought out to test comparative intelligence. They are of two main groups – those which use words in a test, and those which do not. Important among the first type are the Binet–Simon tests, standardised by Terman and others. These tests take the form of questions on general knowledge framed so as to exclude as far as possible the results of formal education, and to reduce environmental differences to as small a factor as possible. A child who answers a set of questions which can usually be answered only by older children is said to have a 'mental age' of those older children, and *vice versa*. A number of these tests have been applied to Whites, Chinese, Japanese, Mexicans, American Indians, and Negroes from the north and the south of the United States. On the results the Whites head the list for intelligence, the Chinese and Japanese come close to them, with the other groups some way behind. Is this a true indication of comparative mental ability? There are reasons for thinking that it is not. Apart from the difficulty of making sure that the command of the language is the same for all the groups, it is probable that the influence of the different types of education has not been fully excluded. Moreover, the different social conditions in

42

which these groups live has probably not allowed the tests to give a fair comparison. Again, these averages are misleading if it is argued from them that all southern Negroes or all American Indians, for instance, are less intelligent than all white people. In each of the groups mentioned there are some people whose score is as high as that of very many white people – higher even than the white average.

After a careful investigation of the results of a great number of these tests, Garth, an American professor of experimental psychology, came to the conclusion that 'differences so far found in the intelligence of races can be easily explained by the influence of nurture and of selection'; that those races which appear from the tests to be inferior have never been properly educated; and that to some extent their low scores are due to their resistance to the European social life by which they are surrounded. This resistance, he said, may not be a sign of inferiority, but the reverse. He says, finally, 'any disposition on our part to withhold from these, or similar, races, because we deem them inferior, the right to a free and full development to which they are entitled must be taken as an indication of rationalisation on account of race prejudice; and such an attitude is inexcusable in an intelligent populace.'

In the present state of our ignorance about comparative mental processes of different races and peoples this is a good working principle to adopt. It may be, however, that more refined analysis will ultimately be able to show that some differences do exist. While there is no unchallengeable evidence for racial inequality of mind there is also no definite proof of identity.

A second type of tests need not use language. This avoids to some extent the difficulty that the subjects tested may not have had the same educational opportunities. And since writing and words are not used in the test, the behaviour of illiterate people and of those who speak different languages can be compared. These tests are alternatively known as performance tests. In some of the best-known examples the people tested have to fit pieces of wood of different shapes into a board with appropriate holes (Goddard–Silvester Form Board); imitate the actions of the investigator in tapping a line of blocks (Knox Cube Test); give appropriate numbers to a series of pictures (Oliver), or trace through a maze with a pencil (Porteus Maze Test).

43

Results from some of these tests have been held to prove that Bantu pupils have a mental age of four to five years below that of white children in Africa. But this is not a clear innate difference. S. Biesheuvel has shown how relatively unfamiliar some of the test objects, such as blocks, jigsaw puzzles, and picture books, were to many Bantu children, and how relatively poor were their homes in other cultural aids. To much of this lack their poor scores could be attributed. Tests on Navaho children have also shown an average rather lower than that for white children, but there was great variation among the Navaho themselves, and this seemed to be definitely linked with the amount of school experience. Practice gained in handling pencils and toys, and in receiving school instruction in situations resembling tests gave some children a definite advantage over others whose early life had been mostly spent in wandering through sage brush herding sheep. Moreover, in such non-verbal tests the less civilised did not always turn out inferior. An anthropologist (Laura Thompson) and a physician (Alice Joseph) working together, found that Hopi children had significantly higher intelligence quotients (mean I.Q. 110 and over) than white children. These Hopi children were highly observant, balanced in mental approach, and very capable of complex and abstract thinking.

One point which seems to emerge from all these performance tests is that differences in language or in education in reading and writing are not the only handicaps in comparing mental ability, and that differences in the kind of social life in which the people concerned have grown up are extremely important, and cannot be overlooked. Not only unfamiliarity with photographs, with pencil and paper, and with the idea of doing a piece of work as quickly as possible, have to be considered. There is also the test situation itself, which is familiar to all school children, but which it not a part of the experience of those who have never gone to school.

What still seem necessary are more tests which will get away from pictures, writing materials, and geometrical shapes, and attempt to measure the ability of people in the practical situations of their everyday life, or in situations based upon their ordinary experience.

The various kinds of projective test devised in recent years suggest some interesting differences in the mentality of people of different cultural groups. These tests are capable of highly sophisticated analysis, but they are still very experimental in their cross-cultural application. So far as they have been pursued, they throw valuable light on individual differences within cultural groups and suggest qualitative differences, as in character structure, between the groups, but they do not give evidence of differences of level of intelligence.

We are now in a position to give some answer to our earlier question about differences in mental capacity and process in different peoples. The results of the great mass of psychological investigation show that on the tests alone the mental ability and intelligence of different racial groups is not the same. From the experiments, some of the African and Amerindian peoples must be placed lower on the scale than western peoples. But for the reasons given these tests must be regarded as inconclusive. In the first place, though the averages for the different racial groups have not been found to be the same, in each group, even in the most primitive, there have emerged individuals whose intelligence and other capacities are of a high order, above the average for that of civilised peoples. Again, the tests are complicated by the fact that in every case the kind of society in which the peoples tested live has determined to a great extent the results obtained. Modes of thinking, the faculty of remembering, the ability to plan, do not exist in a vacuum. All take place in a framework of ideas and practical situations which are different from one society to another. Again, even if the tests could be accepted at face value, they do not enable us to link clearly differences in mentality with differences in skin colour, head form, colour of eyes, etc., or with genetical differences in individuals. In precise terms this is only what *racial* differences in mentality can mean.

If the effects of differences in early training and social environment (cultural differences) could be eliminated, and the constitution and functioning of the mind in different races be determined, there is still the question of whether the results would be found to be qualitative or quantitative. On the qualitative side, it is possible that differences in such fields as musical ability may be found between races. This has not yet been properly investigated. On the quantitative side, it has still to be clearly shown that the moulding influence of social process on the working of the mind can be eliminated from the tests that are applied. But though the experimental basis is small as yet, it does seem from such simple tests as the comparison of similar shapes that the mental functioning of different races is identical.

It has been questioned, by Lucien Lévy-Bruhl and others, whether the mind of a simple nomad or hunter works in the same ways of perception, or uses the same logical processes as does the mind of western industrial man. That different cultural premises affect the structure of argument and its conclusions is agreed. It is also held by some investigators that perception of objects and events is differently structured in different societies. But what the tests of the psychologist and the experiences of the anthropologist seem to show is that whatever differences may exist are qualitative – using different frameworks for selection and classification of sense data – rather than quantitative – having more or less sense perception or power of organisation of sense data. Moreover, the kind of non-rational attitude of man to the external world which Lévy–Bruhl characterised as 'mystic participation' with nature, is not as he thought a hallmark of the mental functioning of 'primitive' peoples but is a feature of some kinds of thought among people in any society anywhere. Peoples of great technological simplicity such as Amazonian hunters or Pacific islands fishermen, despite differences in the way they categorise and express their experience, are apparently not less endowed with mental qualities than their industrial counterparts, or less able to communicate adequately with members of their own or other societies.

What does emerge very clearly from all the work done is the wide gap between the cautious, tentative opinions of the scientist about racial psychology, and the dogmatic views of many ordinary people with a superficial acquaintance with exotic peoples. To say that the 'savage' is inferior in mentality to ourselves, or that he has the mind of a child, indicates the ignorance and prejudice of the speaker. It is absurd at this stage of our knowledge to assert that we have proof that any particular group of people such as the Australian aborigines or South African Bantu, are by the nature of their minds for ever precluded from taking advantage of education, and from reaching that cultural level which we have attained.

This is not to say that people at a low level of technical or economic development should be expected to respond at once to any form of culture which we think good for them. From the very fact of the close relationship between mental process and social life the 'content of the mind' in each 'racial' group is of a specialised kind. As a practical problem it is very necessary to allow for this specialisation. Catchwords like 'assimilation', 'absorption', 'education to white standards', 'raising the cultural level' of a technologically simple community over-simplify the problem. It cannot be assumed that adaptation is an easy process, depending mainly upon the will to adapt. Nor do we know enough about comparative mentality to allow us to shape policy with assurance without further study.

NOTES

1 Such forms of greeting have many variants in different parts of the world, and are an integral part of rituals of communication, with important social overtones. (See: Raymond Firth, 'Verbal and Bodily Rituals of Greeting and Parting', in *The Interpretation of Ritual*, ed. J. S. La Fontaine, London, Tavistock, 1972, 1–38.)
2 *The Times*, 2 July 1974.
3 The following quotation from a letter to the Editor of the *Journal of the Royal African Society*, written by a former member of the Legislative Assembly of (Southern) Rhodesia, is illuminating: 'To deprive settlers, as is being done, of their labour (inefficient and requiring constant supervision and, therefore, dear and not really cheap) is just as honest as to deprive ex-civil servants of their pensions.' (*JRAS*, 1938, 267.)
4 Michael Banton, *Race Relations*, Social Science Paperbacks, London, Tavistock, 1967.
5 See e.g. K. L. Little, *Negroes in Britain*, London, Kegan Paul, 1947; PEP, *Colonial Students in Britain*, London, 1955; Sydney Collins, *Coloured Minorities in Britain*, London, Lutterworth, 1957.
6 George Findlay, *Miscegenation*, Pretoria, 1936.
7 James Weldon Johnson, *Along This Way*, New York, Knopf, 1933, 65, 87–9.

CHAPTER TWO

Man and Nature

If race is not the determinant of human behaviour, where must we look for an explanation? One school of opinion, with a long history, would hold that differences in human ways are primarily due to, or linked with, differences in the natural environment. In various ages Hippocrates, Thucydides, Bodin, Montesquieu, Ratzel, and Huntington have all held in one form or another that the physical qualities of a region, in particular climatic conditions, have worked to shape people's appearance and lives, and to eliminate those who do not conform to the limits set. The phrase, 'the sovereign influence of environment', has summed up the essence of this viewpoint.

But it is now generally agreed, as by Huntington, one of the best-known earlier writers on the subject, that a crude environmentalist theory must fail as an explanation of human differences, and that many other factors than the geographic one must be considered. To realise this one has only to contrast the different ways of life of people in the same environment. The cattle-keeping Hima share Ankole with the agricultural Iru; in Arizona the formerly hunting and col-lecting, and now mainly pastoral Navaho border the flood-farming Hopi; and in the south-east coastal lands of Australia the former hunting, fishing, and foraging aborigines have been succeeded by agricultural, pastoral, and industrial Europeans. As compared with plants and animals Man is helped in attaining relative freedom from his environment by his high degree of mobility, his inventiveness, and his power, especially through the facility of language, of borrowing ideas and applying them to change his condition.

Granted that the rôle of environment is not paramount in deter-mining human culture, what part does it play?

In the first place, the environment in general obviously sets broad limits to the possibilities of human life. Though men have found it possible to survive for short periods at the extremes of the climatic range – up to 29,000 feet on Everest, for instance – no group life has been evolved there. There is no civilisation of the Himalayan peaks. But Man is an ingenious animal. Groups have managed to adapt themselves to very rigorous conditions which at first sight seem impossible for human existence. Small scattered bands of aborigines have lived precariously in the almost waterless deserts of central Australia; Bushmen manage to survive in the Kalahari desert; the Eskimo live in the Arctic wastes. But because of the extreme poverty and harshness of their environment the level of comfort of these peoples has had to remain low, and though they have shown the most remarkable ingenuity and powers of invention, these simple societies have remained until recently, after hundreds or thousands of years, still very much in the grip of their natural surroundings.

In the second place, any specific environment forces to some degree a material way of living upon the people subjected to it. The central Australian aborigines, despite considerable temperature changes, can afford to go naked, and need no solid dwellings; but in traditional conditions their poverty of water, the poor soil, and the spare game and plant life compelled them to lead a wandering, hunting, and foraging life. The Eskimo must have clothing and huts to protect them from the cold and the icy winds, but agriculture is forbidden to them also by the severe conditions. The Hopi, granted their agricultural knowledge, are obliged by the conditions of their desert region to rely not upon immediate rains, but upon flood waters for their maize-growing, and thereby to adopt a system of deep setting and wide spacing of the plants, windbreaks, retaining-walls, and channels to conserve and distribute water, and barriers to prevent erosion of the soil.

Thirdly, the environment, while setting broad limits to human achievement, provides materials for the satisfaction of needs and wants. Granted a desire for clothing, the Eskimo find the stuff for it in the skins of the animals they kill; the Polynesians of the Oceanic islands, without large animals, have vegetable materials to draw upon. And while the Tahitians and other tropical islanders had the bark of the paper mulberry which they could beat into cloth, the Maori of New Zealand, where this tree will not grow, could twine together the fibres of the native flax.

Fourthly, the environment leads to more subtle adaptations in cul-

49

tural life. To mention only religious ritual, the rain-making ceremonies which play so important a part in the agricultural life of the Pueblo Indians of Arizona and New Mexico, and the pastoral life of the Nilotic peoples of the Sudan, are directly related to the conditions of their habitat.

What has been found of the simpler peoples is true also of the advanced peoples of Europe, Asia, and America. Here, too, the geographic factors exercise strong controls upon social life.

Even in simple societies, however, the 'sovereign power of environment' should not be crudely invoked and interpreted.

The geographer and the anthropologist have come to see Man, not as a plastic object on which the environment works its will, but rather, as one geographer has put it, 'a geomorphologic agent', occupying areas of the world not passively, but as an active factor in change. Every people, savage or civilised, has altered its environment to some extent. The aboriginal Australian destroys the vegetation round his water-holes and fires the grass for his hunting; the African agriculturist ravages the forest in his shifting cultivation. The higher civilisations, aided by their superior knowledge, science, and brilliant technology, have harnessed and changed their physical surroundings to a degree where they show little respect for the limitations, and sometimes even the resources of these surroundings. Man-made fields, walls, hedges, and plantations make up the agricultural countryside, which in some areas has suffered serious denudation of timber, and even soil erosion. The sting of the harshest environment has often been drawn; extremes of heat or cold have been overcome or alleviated; poor soils have been enriched; new types of plants have been evolved to meet special climates or resist disease; the lethal effects of fever-ridden tropical swamps have first been checked by the use of quinine and then nullified by draining and choking mosquito breeding-places. Such efforts and achievements go to show that culture rather than environment is paramount.

Between these triumphs of applied science and the achievements of the most lowly developed tribes, the difference is one of degree and not of kind. They, too, have their technology and scientific knowledge, they have their tools, and they are able to face their environment in the confidence that for the most part the balance of power is not all the time against them. Let us examine the type of knowledge they

50

possess. In traditional conditions Australian tribes, for instance, have an extensive natural lore. They know the habits, markings, breeding-grounds, and seasonal fluctuations of all the edible animals, fish, and birds of their hunting grounds. They know the external and some of the less obvious properties of rocks, stones, waxes, gums, plants, fibres, and barks; they know how to make fire; they know how to apply heat to relieve pain, stop bleeding, and to delay the putrefaction of flesh food; and they use also fire and heat to harden some woods and to soften others, and to smooth the insides of dug-out canoes by charring where chipping is no longer possible. They know at least something of the phases of the moon, the movement of tides, the planetary cycles, and the sequence and duration of the seasons; they have correlated together such climatic fluctuations as wind systems, annual patterns of humidity and temperature, and fluxes in the growth and presence of natural species; and when seasonal scarcities or droughts occur they have several lines of retreat from one food to another, from one area to another, from one waterhole to another. In addition they make an intelligent and economical use of the by-products of animals killed for food. The flesh of a kangaroo is eaten; the leg bones are used as fabricators for stone tools and as pins; the sinews become spear bindings; the claws are set into necklaces with wax and fibre; the fat is combined with red ochre as a cosmetic, and the blood is mixed with charcoal as a paint. But in most areas, though the people become cold at night and cluster round fires, they have not found a use for animal skins as covering – perhaps because of the parasites which infest them.

They have some knowledge of simple mechanical principles, and will trim a boomerang again and again to give it the correct curve, or balance a spear in the hand and then cut small portions from the shaft till it bears the correct ratio to the length of the spear-thrower and the thrower's arm. Moreover, on the non-material side, they have built up a social organisation of great complexity, punctuated with rich and dramatic ceremonial observances, and a body of imaginative tales in the form of myths, legends, and religious beliefs.

Now that the general relationship of environment to human be-haviour has been summarily stated, we may examine in more detail the material side of human life.

First let us consider the provision of food, which may be expected

51

to be closely determined by environmental conditions. In every human society food is important from two points of view, the nutritional, satisfying the energy requirements and biological needs of the human body; and the sociological, as a means of expressing and maintaining social relationships. Men do not simply devour food like animals. They make it appetising according to taste, they display it, they serve it, they eat it according to rules, they present it to others, they invite others to meals, they use it as religious offerings. All this causes the processes of body-building and refuelling to be regulated by complex social factors.

One problem of nutrition is that of the quantity of food consumed. On a yearly average, most technologically simple peoples would seem to live above a mere subsistence level. But their food supply is often subject to seasonal variation, which they are unable to remedy by importation from outside, or migration. A severe reduction over a period must affect their output of energy, and Audrey Richards reports of the Bemba of Zambia that for a series of families, studied over a period of eight months, the intake of food was only about 60 per cent of that estimated as adequate for the work that was done. In particular there was a serious shortage of food during the rainy season, when much hoeing had to be done as part of the ordinary agricultural routine. The work was insufficiently done, the productivity of the gardens was lessened, and less ground was put under cultivation than was required. It is not always, however, a matter of simple shortage. The records of M. and S. L. Fortes from the Tallensi of Ghana show that, as with the Bemba, food supplies are at their lowest in the rainy season at the time of greatest agricultural labour. But these people produce a great deal, and have excellent receptacles for storing food, and know how to utilise them. They do not appear to be reckless in the ordinary consumption of food, but they consume and circulate large amounts at harvest festivals. They *could* live sparingly during the dry season where there is less work to be done, and keep their major crop for the wet season, to sustain them in their harder labour. That they do not prefer to do this is due to the social and ritual values they attach to the food, as against the more purely economic and nutritional values.

Another problem of nutrition is the qualitative one. An ordinary human diet to be adequate should have six main components. Three of these are: carbohydrates (sugars and starches), fats, and proteins (complex chemical substances containing nitrogen, and found in all living matter, a typical example being white of egg). These are primarily the fuel stuffs or energy-giving elements. The others are mineral salts (of calcium, iron, etc.), 'accessory' substances (vitamins), and water. These three are not sources of energy, but are important for the building up and functioning of the body.

It is now commonplace in medicine that all of these components are necessary for health, and that a balanced relation should exist between them. Until recent years it was imagined that exotic peoples living a 'natural' life had all that was necessary in their diet, and some back-to-nature movements were even built up on this view. More attention to the matter has now led us to doubt if this is always so. Systematic scientific investigation of the problem indicates that nutritional deficiency can exist among peoples of simple technology in Africa or Oceania, due partly to inadequate natural resources, and partly to inefficient methods of using what is available. But the matter is complicated by various social factors.

There are great variations in the relative amounts of these essential components consumed by many simple hunters and cultivators. In central Australia and other very arid regions the amount of water drunk might seem to be considerably less than that regarded as adequate for bodily functioning. It is possible, however, that these people have made some adjustment to their circumstances by drinking larger quantities at any one time, since it seems that there are no fundamental differences of a physiological kind among these people which allow them to strike a radically different balance of water consumption. An ingenious method of obtaining subsidiary water is used by the central Australians. This consists in digging out from dry river beds and swamps a species of large frog, which has previously filled itself with water in the rainy season, and draining these unfortunate creatures of their fluid reserves.

Many agricultural tribes who live largely on grain or root crops have a high proportion of carbohydrate in their diet, but seem to lack adequate amounts of other essential constituents. The diet of the Bemba, who live largely on millet, is strikingly deficient in fat, and low in animal protein. And though the supply of vitamin C is short, green vegetables are never eaten raw; they are preserved by sun-drying, but this tends to destroy the vitamin. African children living in boarding-schools have been known to refuse for some time to eat green stuff served as salads, saying that they were not mere beasts of the bush. A lack of balance in the opposite direction is seen in the traditional diet of the Eskimo who, living in countries where grain and other plants producing large quantities of starch and sugar are not found, have a very low intake of carbohydrates. They do get some carbohydrates from mosses and berries, and from the blood of the animals which form their principal food. As a whole, they seem to be well nourished and of good physique, and some writers have accordingly concluded that their metabolism is adapted to this situation. It certainly seems that there can be a considerable variation from what the scientist regards as the ordinary dietary standard before deficiency diseases can be medically observed.

It must always be borne in mind, however, that the principal item of diet of, say, an African or Pacific island people is usually supplemented by a number of subsidiary foods, which are often ignored by European observers. The Bemba, for instance, who have little meat, eat caterpillars, locusts, and flying ants, the first being quite an important item of their diet, and containing a high proportion of phosphorus and iron. And as with many African tribes, the native beer is probably a source of vitamin C; it almost certainly contains a considerable amount of vitamin B. The relishes eaten by many agricultural people, again, provide fat and mineral salts, which help to balance their consumption.

In time of hunger many peoples often enlarge the range of their foodstuffs to take in substances ordinarily disregarded.[1] One of the most striking practices is the eating of earth, which occurs in Australia, south-eastern Papua, central America, the Congo, and parts of East Africa. By the casual white observer this practice has been regarded as a quaint custom of dirty savages. But careful observation shows that it is not ordinary mud that is eaten, but special kinds of earth. The Otomac of British Guiana choose from alluvial beds a silty clay which is soft and smooth; the Australians of the Daly River do likewise, digging it out from underneath the slopes of the river bank; they also eat the dry earth of the termite ant-hills, a practice followed also in parts of West Africa. This eating of earth is not simply a means of filling the belly. Edible earths contain a high proportion of mineral salts, so that whether the people realise it nor not, they obtain therefrom essential constituents for bodily health. This is clearly shown by a series of analyses of edible earths from Kenya, Tanzania, and Nigeria. It is probably significant from this point of view that in some tribes, such as the Bemba, earth-eating is practised mainly by pregnant women and young children. The contributions to the diet made by these often unconsidered items may be extremely important when a simple hunting or cultivating people in contact with civilisation are changing their food supplies, or when an attempt is being made to improve their dietary position.

It must be remembered again that the consumption of an apparently similar foodstuff by two tribes may not mean that the nutritional constituents are identical. Orr and Gilks found that the diet of the Kikuyu of Kenya, who live largely on white millet and maize, was deficient in calcium. The diet of the Bemba, who live largely on another species of millet, is very similar. But the finger millet of the Bemba contains about sixteen times as much calcium as the white millet of the Kikuyu, and bone deformations among the Bemba are thus much less probable.

On the whole, then, it is clear that the factors of the physical environment play an important part in regulating the food supply of a people, especially on the qualitative side, and may have striking results on their health and physique.

But to a considerable extent social factors influence the situation. Many peoples, African or Oceanian as well as western, do not use their resources to the full because of some particular dietetic theory. Just as to us bread is the 'staff of life', so to many native peoples one particular food is the staple. To the Polynesian Tikopia of the Solomon Islands the staple is the taro, a root somewhat like a potato, which they call 'the basis of food'. To many Africans it is millet porridge. The Tallensi of Ghana say, 'Porridge is food, it makes you strong. But if you eat too much of other things they spoil your belly.' And they only feel satisfied when they have eaten about a pound and a half of it at a sitting. When a root crop is in season it is cooked instead of porridge, not to avoid monotony, but to make the grain last longer. Meat is not food as porridge is; it is 'gluttony'. The Bemba of Zambia say that there is only one true food, porridge. After a dish of sweet potatoes or maize cobs a Bemba may declare that he has had nothing to eat all day! Both these peoples eat a soup or stew of vegetables with meat if they have it, as a relish with the porridge. This soup provides necessary elements for their nutriment, but they look upon it as giving flavour rather than as real food. So important is the relish that without it a housewife will often not cook porridge for her family. Before attempting to improve a local diet it is essential, then, to understand the local theories on the subject.

Indifference, aesthetic aversion to some kinds of food, or traditional taboos may also be important. The Andamanese do not trap animals or birds, though they could easily do so; the Tikopia do not eat many kinds of birds, or eels, for religious reasons, though their Polynesian cousins, the Maori, eat both freely, and prize the flesh and fat that they yield. The complexity of taste and taboos in food is seen further in the Tikopia attitude towards a deep-sea shark. Some of these people refuse to eat this shark because it eats man, others do eat it and say they are taking revenge because of its man-eating habits. Both the Andamanese and the Tikopia have other sources of flesh food, so that they do not suffer. But among the Tallensi of West Africa, though meat is a great delicacy, and a medium-sized guinea-fowl may last a family of seven about a week, some other kinds of flesh food are barred. Women never cook or eat domestic fowls or dogs, which are common. Hyenas, though killed by young men, are spurned by them as filthy things which dig up and devour corpses, though old men consider them a luxury. In many tribes, again, funeral taboos bar the close kinsfolk of the dead from eating the best kinds of food for long periods. All this has analogy in western culture. Europeans normally do not have funeral taboos about food. But they do have a taboo against eating domestic dogs and cats, though not against eating domestic fowls or rabbits – unless they have been special pets. In all cultures such individual and group attitudes may affect the amount of animal fat and protein consumed.

Economic conditions, again, may influence the nutritional balance. The poorer people in many districts of Sri Lanka, for instance, according to Nicholls, do not milk their cows, but keep them for breeding cart bulls, the manure they produce for the fields, and the price they fetch from the butcher. From rough calculation he estimated that only about twenty million gallons of milk from cows and buffalo were available for consumption per annum among five and a

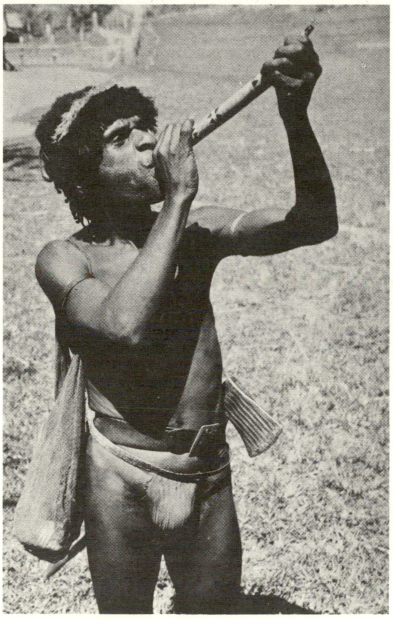

1 Smoking from a bamboo pipe, Tapini, New Guinea *(By courtesy of the Royal Society of Arts)*

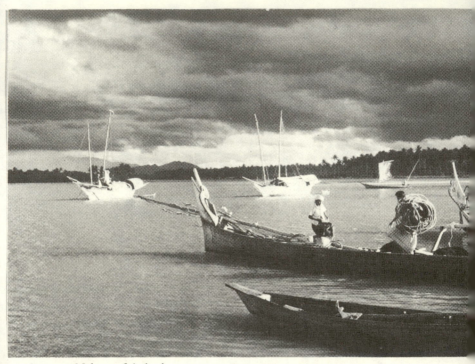

2 Malay craft in harbour

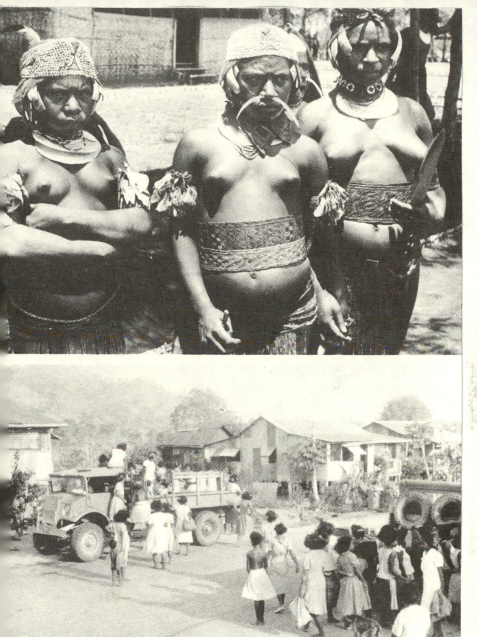

3 *Above:* Young women of Minj, New Guinea highlands, in traditional dress

4 *Below:* Farewelling a women's visiting cricket team, Kilakila, Papua

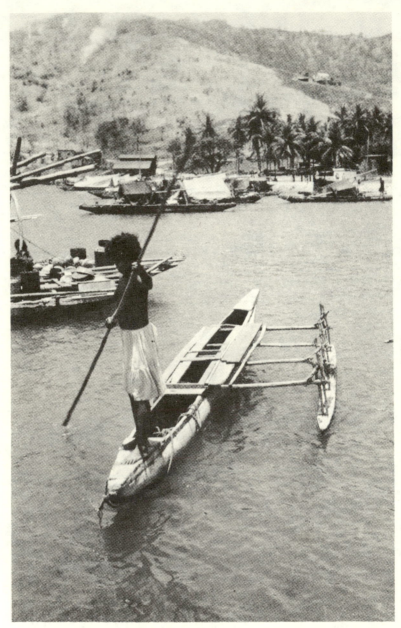

5 Outrigger canoe being poled, Port Moresby

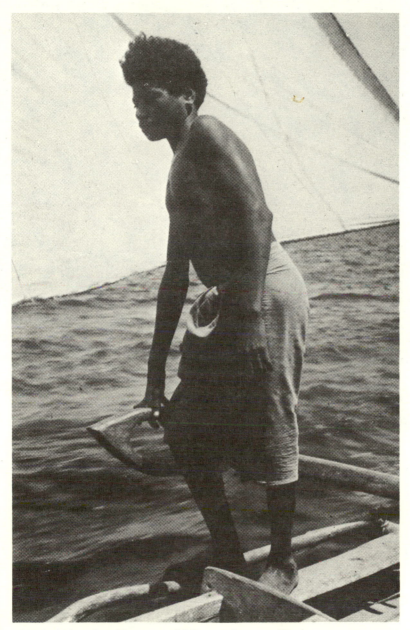

6 At the helm of a sailing canoe, Mailu, south coast of Papua

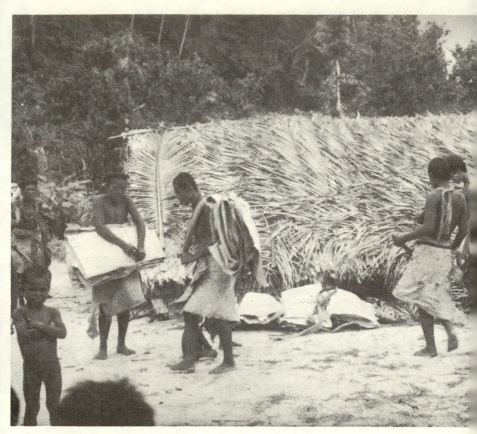
7 Bark-cloth payment for canoe builders, Tikopia

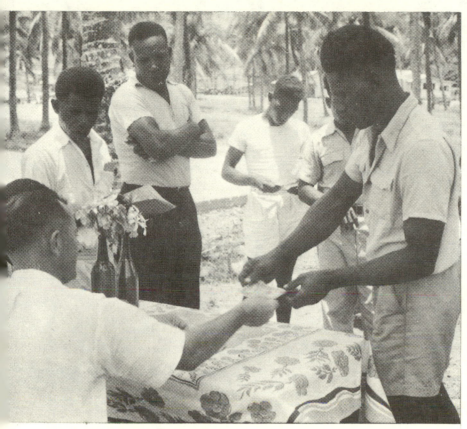

8 Contribution to co-operative purchase of trading schooner, Toaripi Association in Port Moresby, Papua

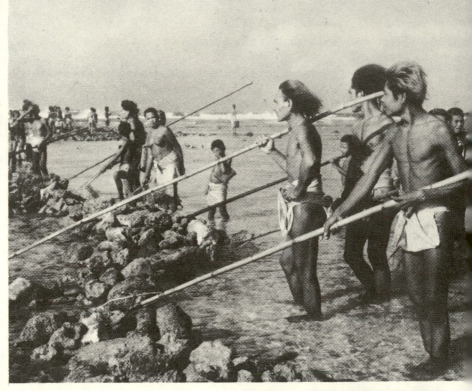

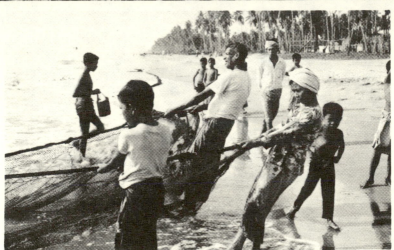

9 *Above :* Fish drive on reef, Tikopia

10 *Below :* Hauling in seine on Kelantan beach, Malaysia

half million people. Yet milk would be a most valuable addition to the diet of the poor.

On the other hand, deficiencies in local food resources may be overcome by trade with other communities. A well-known example here is the extensive trade in salt, which is carried freely over central Africa, and helps to supplement the diet of many people.

The contact of non-industrial peoples with the results of western technology has both given possibilities of remedying nutritional deficiences and created new food problems. Scientific research, by the analysis of diets, by the study of nutritional diseases, by showing ways of increasing soil fertility and reducing erosion, and by suggesting new types of food for cultivation, can do much to remedy food deficiences. Indirectly it may help by showing the relation of diets to local custom, to division of labour between the sexes, to economic organisation, to theories of taste, and to religious taboos. Changes in the food supply cannot be made without taking these social factors into consideration, and a proper anthropological study may be able to point out new types of food which are best adapted to the local social conditions, and the way in which these new foods can best be worked into the local system of life. But the advent of industrial civilisation is apt also to create fresh problems. Changes in the economic life of the people, ill-considered regulations about the preservation of game, or the abandonment of beer-drinking, may cause a degeneration of their diet at first unperceived. Here also careful study is necessary in order to see that the sufferer is not put in a worse position by our well-meant efforts to improve him.

Since the securing of food is basic to every human society, the methods used have been taken for the classification of societies into a number of broad types. These general types are:

1 Food-gatherers, hunters, and fishers.
2 Pastoralists.
3 Agriculturists.
4 Artisans.

These broad types can be split up into a number of sub-types. Some people in the first type, like the Eskimo, are mainly hunters and fishers, others, like the Negritos of Malaya, or some of the Californian Indians, are largely food-gatherers. The most important division among the agriculturists is made according to the technical methods and implements employed: first, those peoples who use for cultivation a simple digging stick: second, those who use a form of hoe; third, those who use the plough. Within these divisions there are still further sub-types. In olden days the Maori of New Zealand used a digging-stick which they had adapted as a form of spade by fixing on the front a wooden tread. This implement was used not by pressure at the side as in a European spade, but by reaching the foot round to the front. Again, this method of classifying societies does not mean an exclusive separation of them. Many simple agriculturists hunt wild animals, catch fish, and forage for forest foods. Many pastoralists practise a simple form of agriculture as well; and the use of the plough usually involves animal traction and some degree of pastoralism. This classification, then, which does give a convenient frame of reference, refers only to the major occupation, technique, and food-producing mechanisms of the people concerned.

Until recently students of human culture were interested in this classification primarily from the point of view of establishing the evolution of societies. They attempted to show how from the simplest hunting and collecting stages mankind had developed the more complex agricultural and industrial occupations. Now, however, although the evolution of the more complex from the simpler forms is not denied as a general process, it is seen that the process has by no means been identical in every case, and attention is directed mainly to the examination of the particular kind of social life associated with each type of food production.

Our analysis of the food problem among technically undeveloped peoples has shown that they have considerable knowledge of their natural environment, that they have ingenious techniques for solving their problems, and that they have a material apparatus, however simple, through which this knowledge and technique is applied. In this connection certain problems spring to mind. How far are their knowledge, technique, and material apparatus a direct response to their environmental conditions? How far have they shown a capacity for invention? How far have they adopted ideas from other peoples? How far do they rely upon traditional forms and the lines laid down by custom? Our answer may be exemplified, first, by a brief reference to some aspects of East African native agriculture, and, secondly, by an analysis of some principles of canoe construction in Polynesia.

The Ecological Survey of Zambia (formerly Northern Rhodesia) published in 1937 a valuable exhaustive study of the soils, vegetation, and agricultural systems of the north-west of the territory. This has shown how climatic differences and the processes of physiographic change have determined the main soil classes of the area, and how these together have determined the different types of vegetation. This close correlation between vegetation and soil type is widely understood and used by the Africans, who adapt their agricultural methods to the type of woodland or grassland cover which the soil carries. They know what kind of crop each soil will best take, and how long before its potentialities will be exhausted. By reference to the predominant vegetation it has been possible to distinguish a number of main agricultural systems in the area, such as the Woodland system, the Grassland system, the Thorn system, and the Thicket system, with sub-types of each. It will be sufficient to discuss only two of these here: the Northern Plateau system, of the Woodland type, and the Central Kalahari Plains system, of the Grassland type.

The agricultural system of the Northern Plateau tribes is based on the traditional method known as *chitemene*. This consists of felling trees over a larger area than that to be cultivated, lopping the branches off, and carrying them with their leaves into low stacks or piles, which are then burned. The result is to destroy weeds and to leave a thick patch of ash into which the seed is sown, either with or without subsequent hoeing. The main crop is kaffir corn or finger millet. On the unburnt land cassava or sweet potatoes may be planted in mounds. In the simplest form of this *chitemene* cultivation, practised by the eastern Kaonde, the garden is abandoned after three years and a fresh site chosen; in more elaborate forms a block of land may be so worked up to six years. On the whole, the land is of low productivity.

In the Central Kalahari Plains system bush cultivation is not an essential element, and agriculture is based upon grassland gardening. There is a variety of soils, in most of which moisture is conserved in the lower horizons to a varying degree, and there is a close relationship between the different garden types used and the soil and moisture

59

variations of the different zones of grasslands. These garden types are employed, moreover, by each tribe in different combination according to locality.

Seven principal types of garden have been recognised in the area: the raised garden for maize and kaffir corn; the ridge garden for root crops; the dry village garden for mixed crops; the moist village seepage garden for mixed crops; the drained seepage garden for winter-planted maize, taro, etc.; the lagoon garden for winter-planted maize, and the riverbank garden for winter-planted maize. The sites for these different types of garden are decided with the help of 'indicator grasses', which by their nature and growth reveal the possibilities of the soil. Among the Lozi tribe these grasses appear to have been formed into a traditional reference list. In contrast to the *chitemene* system of shifting cultivation, the last five of these garden types allow of practically indefinite cultivation, and even the first two, by exchange of mound and trench, and by long fallowing, may be worked on a rotation system.

Here, then, we see a very close response of the African to the environmental conditions, and the exercise of considerable ingenuity in making use of the resources thus presented. But environmentalism is not the whole story.

In the first place, as the Ecological Survey itself shows, there has been considerable borrowing of ideas by one tribe from another. The raised garden, the ridge garden, and the village garden for mixed crops have all been adopted to some extent from the Sikololo-speaking tribes by immigrant tribes from Angola. But, on the other hand, they have not adopted the drained seepage garden and the lagoon garden, although they frequently occupy sites suitable for the cultivation of winter-planted maize, for which these garden types would be eminently appropriate. The survey, in fact, often noted the neglect of good land of this type by the Angolan tribes. To what is this neglect due? The answer seems to lie in the weight of their tradition, a conservative force which, while often of the utmost value, can at times impede a more efficient adaptation, or at least bend choice in one direction when alternatives are possible.

The particular agricultural technique adopted may also depend upon other cultural factors: the availability of new implements such as the plough; the entry of new factors into the economic organisation such as a market for commercial crops, or a demand for male labour in European industry, or the introduction of foreign plants. All of these factors are now tending to change African agriculture.

We may now turn to consider the same problems in regard to the Polynesian canoe. The Polynesian people live on islands widely scattered over a great area of the Pacific Ocean. Some of these islands are low coral atolls, others are ancient volcanic peaks with more or less low land around. Agriculture and fishing are the two principal methods of obtaining food, and all these people are daring navigators with traditions of oversea voyaging. As cultivated plants they have bread-fruit, taro, yam, coconut, sweet potato, banana, and sugar cane; they draw in addition upon a variety of forest fruits which grow wild. In all the islands there are timber trees used for the construction of canoes, though the kind, size, and quality of the woods available vary considerably from one island to another. Before the days of European contact they worked these timbers with implements of stone and shell. They had no metals, though it is argued by a few anthropologists that they once knew the arts of metal working. For cordage they had in New Zealand the fibres of the native flax, a plant with swordlike leaves, and elsewhere the fibres of hibiscus and coconut.

Incidentally, the coconut palm (which is not found in New Zealand) provides a great variety of objects. From its fronds are made roof thatch, floor-mats, baskets, fans, and, when dried, torches for fishing. From the ribs of the leaves are made food-pounders, stirrers, and tongs. The nuts provide drink when green, and food of various kinds when more mature; empty, they give water bottles, or if small, lime containers. From pieces of the shell cups are made to hold kava or tattooing pigment; graters for sago-making or preparing coconut shavings; or beads. The fibrous material which sheaths the leaf-base is used to make bags or strainers, and the fibre from the green nuts is prepared as cordage of many types. The trunk itself yields diggingsticks, poles, and sometimes even heavier timbers. From the variety of uses made of the coconut alone it will be seen that the Polynesians have tackled with ability the resources which their environment presents.

The need for canoes in Polynesia is primarily an economic one. They are essential for catching large fish beyond the confines of the shore reef, and they serve the needs of transport and travel partly around the coast and partly to other islands. But it would be a mistake to look upon the canoe simply as a material adjunct to Polynesian life. It is a focus for the economic organisation of the people in that its building demands co-operation for log-hauling and working the timbers, and its use means also co-operative effort. It is an object of ownership, highly valued, and needing payment for its timbers and for the skill of its construction. It is an object of inheritance also. Traditionally, it has frequently had a religious aspect, as when it is dedicated to the gods, or when the tools used in its building are believed to owe their efficiency to spiritual power. Related to this is the taboo which is frequently imposed upon women to prevent them from entering canoes. Again, it is mentioned frequently in the traditional tales of the people; it is the vehicle by which their ancestors, and sometimes their gods too, arrived at their present island home. It often has a name of its own, and this name bears with it all kinds of historical and legendary associations. It is highly valued, not only from the utilitarian point of view; it serves the expression of deep emotions, as when it is dedicated to decay at the death of a chief or broken at the death of a sister's child. Finally, it is an object of aesthetic interest, and on it is frequently lavished a wealth of wood-carving and ornament. We are concerned here with its structure in relation to the economic needs which it serves, and with the way in which human ingenuity has constructed it from the materials offered by the environment. But the wider social considerations should be borne in mind, since without them one cannot explain much of the behaviour of the people in using their vessel.

Apart from simple means such as floats or rafts Polynesian craft are of three types: the single canoe, the double canoe, and the single outrigger canoe. Sometimes these types can be found in the same area, though in most of the islands the coming of European civilisation has caused certain of the larger and more complicated ones, especially the double canoe, to be discarded. But, in general, throughout central Polynesia the canoe with the single outrigger is still in use. This is the type which I propose to discuss (cf. Plate 5).

The first obvious requirement of a canoe is buoyancy and seaworthiness. There are three kinds of construction in use in Polynesia to meet this end. One is the simple dug-out in which the trunk of a tree is hollowed out and used as a hull of the vessel without further building up. The suitability of the craft for work at sea is then governed by the size of timber available, and as many Polynesian islands do not produce huge tree trunks, such a simple dug-out hull can be used only on a lake or river or within a protecting reef. For work at sea the hull must be raised and an extra plank lashed as a washstrake on either side. Where the timber obtainable is small, even this method is not adequate, and the canoe must be built up in sections or from a series of planks laid down on a keel. In Aitutaki the hull of a vessel is made of one, two, or three pieces, according to the length of timber available. But environmental considerations are not always solely responsible for this. In the Society Islands there were three types of craft. The simple dug-out, with a thin strap along the upper margin of the hull to form a small gunwale, was used for fishing on and near the reef. A larger canoe called *va'a*, round-bottomed, had a hull of a dug-out to which were added washstrakes and bow and stern covers. These were used singly with an outrigger for ordinary sea work, or lashed together as a double canoe for ceremonial use or to carry a war party. In the Leeward Islands of this group another type of vessel called *pahi* was in use. It was about fifty feet in length, and built up of small planks on a keel. This difference in type of the *pahi* from the *va'a* was partly due to the absence from the Leeward Islands of the large trees suitable for making a hull out of a single trunk. But it was due also to the perception of the value of the different technique. Though built of small pieces of wood the *pahi* were much superior in strength, convenience, and seaworthiness to the *va'a.*

In ancient Polynesia metal nails could not be used in canoe building, and the pieces of the craft were lashed together with strong cordage. Even nowadays this method is still common. The method of lashing the washstrake to the hull of the craft differs considerably from one island group to another, and cannot be dictated by purely environmental considerations. Figure 1 (*a*) shows the main varieties of this attachment. It will be seen that they differ considerably in technical efficiency, that is, in not admitting water through the joint, and in withstanding the impact of the waves. Rarely is the washstrake simply laid on top of the edge of the hull and lashed, though this is done in Tokelau, in Aitutaki, and for part of the timber's length, in

Ra'iatea. The three main ways of dealing with the problem are: laying battens over the joint on one or both sides and lashing round them; leaving a flange on the inside of the washstrake and of the hull, and lashing through the flange; and overlapping strake and hull by thinning down one or the other. The use of flanges on the timbers – as in Samoa and Tikopia – means that no holes at all appear on the outside of the vessel. Unless, however, the flange is wide and strong, there is some danger of the joint weakening with the battering of the waves. The most efficient method of attachment would seem to be that of Manihiki and Rakahanga, which uses both flange and batten, and where no lashing appears on the outer surface of the vessel. We have no evidence as to the precise origination of each of these varying types of attachment, but from their distribution over the various island groups, and on the other hand their individuality as between islands which have had communication, it is clear that processes of local invention and of adaptation of technique have both played their part.

The next requirement which the canoe has to meet is that of stability. The Maori craft, where huge tree trunks five feet or more in diameter were available, were single hulls with no other support. But this was not possible in most of the other Polynesian islands. Hence the outrigger, which was almost essential for any free use of the canoe far at sea. The single outrigger consists of a float of light wood some distance out from the hull and attached to it by a number of poles or booms. Here comes in a secondary technical problem. The great difference in diameter of the hull and of the float means that they do not displace the same amount of water, and that therefore the former is much higher above the surface than the latter. There must be, then, some device which will keep the canoe level (Fig. 1 (b)). One means of meeting the problem is to curve the outrigger booms; another is to keep the booms straight, but maintain the float at a distance from them by connecting pegs. The former gives what is called 'direct attachment', the latter 'indirect attachment'. The value of the indirect attachment is that it gives a level platform of booms, and does away with the necessity of finding timbers of the right curvature. It is the most common method adopted in Polynesia. The canoes of Hawaii, however, use a direct attachment, and some canoes of Rarotonga and Samoa use a branched boom which is in essence the same. Fish-

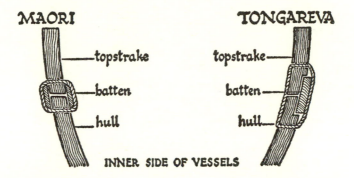

MAORI

—topstrake

—batten

—hull

TONGAREVA

topstrake—

batten—

hull—

INNER SIDE OF VESSELS

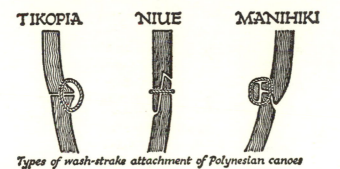

TIKOPIA

NIUE

MANIHIKI

Types of wash-strake attachment of Polynesian canoes

Fig. 1 (*a*) – Technique of Polynesian canoe-building

65

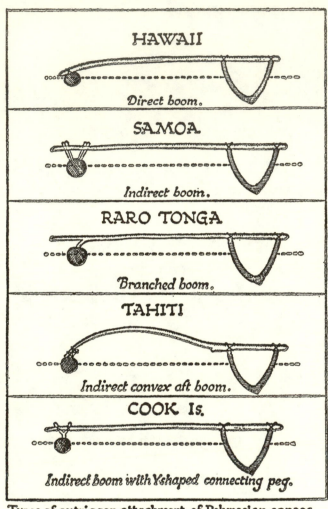

HAWAII
Direct boom.

SAMOA
Indirect boom.

RARO TONGA
Branched boom.

TAHITI
Indirect convex aft boom.

COOK Is.
Indirect boom with Y shaped connecting peg.

Types of outrigger attachment of Polynesian canoes.

Fig. 1 (*b*) – Technique of Polynesian canoe-building
(After P. H. Buck)

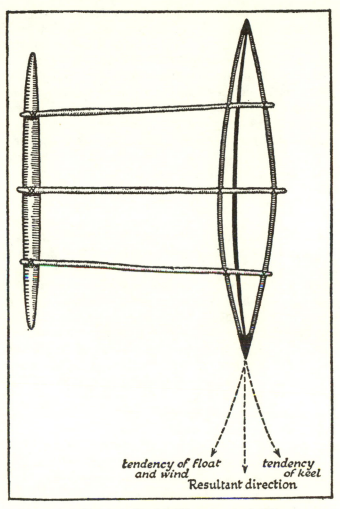

tendency of float
and wind

tendency
of keel

Resultant direction

Fig. 1 (c)—Technique of Gilbertese canoe-building
(After A. Grimble)

ing canoes of Tahiti have the fore-boom stout and stiff, and attached to the float by pegs, but the after-boom is a slender branch which describes a wide curve, and is lashed directly to the float. These canoes are often sailed, with the outrigger always to windwards. The advantage of the slender after-boom is that, being pliant, it trails longer on the surface of the water when a sudden squall strikes the sail, and so allows the crew more time to throw their weight on the outrigger and prevent a capsize. Moreover, even when the canoe is not sailed, it is said that the pliant afterboom makes the craft ride more smoothly over the waves. This device has, however, not been generally adopted, though in recent times it has been taken over by the people of Rapa and those of Fakarava in the Tuamotu group.

There are many local variations of the indirect type of attachment. Straight pegs, bent pegs, branched pegs, and U-shaped pegs are used, generally in pairs, as also Y-shaped pegs, in different islands. These are usually driven into the soft wood of the float, and the tops of the booms lashed to them. To strengthen the attachment when the canoe is lifted, or battered by heavy seas, a subsidiary lashing of stout cord often connects float to boom as well. The style of this lashing often varies in an interesting way according to the type of the canoe, and the circumstances in which it is used. The lower part of the cord sometimes passes right round the float, which is the easiest way of securing it. But if the craft has to be dragged about a great deal among the coral reefs with which these waters abound, then the cord will soon be chafed through, and a better way is to run it through a hole bored in the upper part of the float. For ordinary Samoan canoes, which are used for fishing in shallow reef waters, the cord is run through such a hole. But for the canoe which is used in catching bonito, which are pursued in shoals in the open sea, the lashing is passed round the float. This is possible, since the craft has to be light to give it speed in the chase, and it can be carried down to the water and not dragged. In Tikopia, on the other hand, all canoes have the lashing passed round the float. The reason is that the reef round this island is very narrow, and with a little care the float need not be scraped on the coral. Hence the delicate work of boring the float is avoided. Here, then, the type of suspensory lashing is seen to be a function of several factors: a need for efficiency in a firm outrigger; skill in the work of boring a float; care of property in avoiding damage to the lashing; and the particular situation in which the canoe is to be used.

In general we see also that the adoption of a particular solution to one technical problem – in this case the adoption of an outrigger for stability – immediately raises other problems – in this case of maintenance of the equilibrium of the vessel and the solidity of its attachments. And in each case local circumstances and local ingenuity have been at work within the same broad framework of ideas.

Only one further requirement of the canoe can be discussed here, namely, its steadiness and response to control. The drag of the single outrigger on one side of the canoe hull inevitably affects the propulsion and steering of the vessel, which if left to itself would gradually work round in a circle. Most Polynesian canoes – making allowance for modern degeneration – can be either paddled or sailed (a few are poled when there is much shallow reef water). It is interesting to observe that the outrigger is not set indifferently either to starboard or port, but is nearly always on the port side, leaving the starboard side free for a right-handed man to work his paddle. Occasionally it is set to starboard side for a left-handed man. But even here local custom comes in to complicate efficiency, since in the Marquesas and Napuka in the Tuamotu group it seems to have been the fashion to have it to starboard, and it is incredible that every man in these islands should have been left-handed.

The Polynesians are expert canoemen, and can ply the paddle and steer effectively from the one side only; I remember how I was laughed at when I first acquired a Tikopia canoe and started to paddle it by dipping alternately on each side. But they are not content to have to counteract the drag of the outrigger by human force alone. In some islands at least the canoe-builders have seen the technical difficulty, and to a large measure overcome it. In the first place they have made the hull of the craft asymmetrical in cross-section, broadening the side next to the outrigger, and steepening that away from the outrigger. The result is that when the craft is propelled the tendency of the hull by itself is to veer away from the direct line in a curve opposite to the pull of the outrigger. This pull is thus to a large extent neutralised. Secondly, they build the canoe with a special keel either with deflected sections, or curved with the convex side towards the outrigger. Here, again, when the craft is in motion the tendency is for the hull by itself to curve away from the pull of the outrigger. The result is that the two tendencies largely neutralise each other, and the canoe proceeds on a straight course (see Fig. 1 (c), giving a diagram of an analogous Gilbertese type from the neighbouring area of Micronesia).

Our examination of the Polynesian outrigger canoe has shown that while environment has dictated the form of the vessel and the technical methods used to a considerable extent, human invention has effectively been able to overcome the difficulties encountered. Moreover, while custom and tradition have guided the procedure of the craftsman, he must have often borrowed ideas fom other islands and applied them to the solution of his local problems.

Even in a technically primitive society such as that of Congo pygmies or Australian aborigines, we are not dealing with the mind of an unintelligent being, nor of one ruled rigidly by the conditions of his physical surroundings. We are dealing with the mind of a man with a definite system of knowledge and technique, adaptable, willing to learn, and capable of profiting by the lessons of experience.

NOTES

1 The economic and social reactions of a Polynesian people to famine are described in my book *Social Change in Tikopia*, London, Allen & Unwin, 1959, 51–76.

CHAPTER THREE

Work and Wealth of Primitive Communities

THE eager extension of our western industrial system over the world, with its desire for raw materials, for new markets, and for fresh sources of labour supply, has brought us into contact with the economic attitudes of many alien peoples. The white man in the tropics often finds these difficult to understand. He encounters resistance to his plans for economic expansion and social betterment from what he often thinks are inadequate and irrational local ideas. In the Trobriand Islands men often refused to dive for pearl-shell for a trader and went out on a fishing expedition instead, even though they could earn ten or twenty times more from the first than from the second. A man of the Solomon Islands could formerly buy three sticks of tobacco for a shilling, but he might prefer those three sticks in exchange for his wares to two shillings in money. In New Guinea and elsewhere the wages earned by months of labour may be dissipated in a few days by gifts to kinsfolk and the purchase of paltry trinkets. In East and South Africa, where cattle-keeping is an important part of tribal life, the African may hang on to the most decrepit beasts and overstock his pastures to the peril of their fertility in an obviously uneconomical way. How can these facts be explained? Have we to do with people who have no sense of value and of economic principles? Observations such as these, which could be paralleled from almost any part of Africa or Oceania, and from various other regions as well, have led to a number of popular misconceptions about local behaviour and the fundamental motives which govern it.

It should be the function of the anthropologist, whose business is the systematic study of exotic communities, to throw light on these problems. Unfortunately, however, many anthropological observations on economics have been studies of technology and arts and crafts, rather than of the basic principles which control the work and wealth of pre-industrial or pre-capitalist societies.

Economics is the study of that broad aspect of human activity which is concerned with resources, their limitations and uses, and the organisation whereby they are brought into relation with human wants. In modern industrial societies economists have worked out an elaborate technique for the study of this organisation, and have produced a body of generalisations upon it. It is still a matter of argument as to how far this technique and these generalisations can be applied in the study of non-industrial communities. These communities have a comparatively simple material equipment which has not been integrated into an industrial organisation. They are frequently small in size, and they lack any system of wide inter-communication with each other – they are not part of a world market. Moreover, apart from their contact with western civilisation, they may lack that price system which can act, however imperfectly, as a measure of wants and energies. The economist, again, assumes in his analysis certain basic human attitudes which he refers ultimately to his experience of what people do in our society. It is possible that these attitudes are not present with the same force in non-industrial people, and that other attitudes may take their place as the prime regulators of human behaviour. For all these reasons some of the terms which the modern economist uses – such as capital, saving, and interest – cannot be applied directly in economic anthropology.

Certain broad principles, however, do seem to emerge from our studies. It has been said by an earlier German economist that some primitive peoples are in a kind of pre-economic stage in which an individual search for food is the characteristic feature. Nowadays this would not be admitted. In every human group there is a problem of food supply in relation to population, and this problem is not one realised by single individuals in isolation, but is dealt with as a collective question by some planned system of production and distribution. It is important for us to understand from the outset that family ties, wider obligations to kinsfolk and to neighbours, loyalty to chiefs and elders, respect for clan taboos and beliefs in control of food and other things by spirits, ancestors, and gods can all play their part in this system.

How do people work in their own tribal life when they are not subject to the regulations of a European employer? They do not have a wage system, in which so much reward is given for so much

72

labour. Participation in work is often undertaken as a duty towards the person who wants the work done, rather than for the material gain which can be expected from him. But work for its own sake is not regarded as a duty. There are no sayings like, 'Satan finds mischief for idle hands to do', or moral ideas about the 'dignity of labour'. And time is not such an important element in the economic process as it is with us. The calculation of payment for work is not made on the basis of the units of time spent by the different persons engaged, and if there is a pause between two steps of the task – as in waiting for a metal or a liquid to heat up, or cloth to dry, or shoots to sprout – there is no feeling that the time taken is 'lost' or 'wasted', just because of this. It is perhaps difficult for the European reader to understand just how much moral value he himself unconsciously gives to the passing of time, and how little an African attaches to it. This does not mean that Africans are normally idle, or slack at what they are supposed to be doing. When the work itself calls for industry, or even haste, they respond, but this response is always within the sphere of the needs of the task; again, they frequently find other occupations for their spare time. But a general responsibility to be busy does not lie on them.

It is sometimes imagined that the main drive to the economic activity of a tribal people is their immediate desire to satisfy their material wants. It will be obvious from what has been said in the last chapter that this is an important factor in their life. But it would be untrue to interpret their economic organisation as a simple response to their requirements of food, clothing, shelter, and the like. In the first place, it is a socialised and not an individual response. The values which they put upon their food do not consist simply in its capacity to satisfy hunger, but in the use they can make of it to express their obligations to their relatives-in-law, their chiefs, their ancestors; to show their hospitality; to display their wealth; to initiate or marry off their sons. The value that is put on a canoe is not to be measured only in terms of the capacity of the vessel to carry goods and passengers, and of the fish that are caught from it, but also by the way in which it is a symbol of craftsmanship in wood, an object of artistic carving and decoration, a reminder of traditional voyages, and even the resting-place or embodiment of a god. The value of a cow does not simply consist in its yield of milk, and the uses to which its flesh, hide, and horns can be put, or in what it will fetch at a sale, but also in its rôle as part of a marriage portion, as a ritual sacrifice, and as a token of social status. The whole economic system of the people is run with this complex set of values in mind. From this it is seen, then, in the second place, that many of the wants upon which their economic life is based are of an immaterial kind. And the desire to build up a reputation may lead a man to accumulate more food, or cows, or canoes; but in some cases it leads him to reject mere accumulation – deliberately to give more than he receives in an exchange; or to expend his resources in marrying off his son, or burying his father; or, in the extreme case of the potlatch of the American Indian of the north-west coast, in destroying his most valued property in order to outface a rival in public esteem. This is all economic behaviour, in that it involves his making a choice as to what he will do with his wealth. But it is not covered by the idea that the maximisation of *material* satisfactions is the economic goal.

Again, it is not an immediate return that is always sought. As Malinowski and Thurnwald have shown, the principle of reciprocity seems to be fundamental to most human relationships. When, as often happens in a non-industrial society, a present is made or a service given without any payment handed over on the spot what has been given is mentally 'chalked up' by both parties, and ultimately a return is made. It may be of the same type, or of a different type; it may take the form of material goods or labour, or of some action as wailing at a funeral, or a public recital in praise of the donor. Sometimes there is an immediate response. In Tikopia, when one man at a dance festival chants a song in honour of another man, the latter at once trails out before the assembly a length of barkcloth and presents it to him to 'cover' the song. But for a funeral there is an element of de-layed response. A kinsman of the dead person is not supposed to pre-pare his own food, since his heart is heavy with mourning; he is accordingly fed by some one else who comes in from outside for the purpose, moved by 'sympathy', as the Tikopia say. At the end of three days the mourner hands over to his 'feeder' a wooden bowl, some sinnet cord, and some fish-hooks as payment. But when next there is a funeral in the family of the other, he himself returns the service, going along with his basket of food, and receiving similar property in return. The two sets of acts thus cancel each other out,

74

This example illustrates other points: how closely the preparation and eating of food is connected with sentiments of sympathy and family affection; and how the principle of reciprocity demands not merely that property should be handed over in return for food, but that the service of sympathy should itself receive acknowledgment and return.

To what is all this complex behaviour due? Alfred Marshall has said that 'in the ruder stages of human life many of the services rendered by the individual to others are nearly as much due to hereditary habit and unreasoning impulse, as are those of the bees and ants'.[1] It is true that he goes on at once to qualify this by saying that a deliberate sense of self-sacrifice and tribal duty soon make their appearance. But it is important to realise that the habit is not hereditary, nor the impulse unreasoning, but the result of training in the social values of the particular community; and, as we have just seen, that self-sacrifice and duty are not intelligible until they are considered in relation to the demand for reciprocity.

Continuing our summary observations on this kind of economic system, we see that it is not characterised by any permanent specialisation of individuals or groups in different tasks. Sometimes, as with the metal-workers of Africa, a man or a family will devote their major interest to a specific task, but even here they have, as a rule, some subsidiary source of income. In an Oceanic island every man is normally a cultivator and a fisherman, and has some competence in woodworking, manufacture of thatch and cordage, and all the other crafts practised in the community. There is division of labour, particularly between the sexes, but no one is expected to gain his livelihood by the exercise of one special skill alone. An obvious result of this is the absence of much seasonal unemployment, and of a floating labour supply which depends upon capitalist initiative for its subsistence.

Work in co-operation is a frequent aspect of non-industrial economic life. The stimuli which keep the working group together may be different from those we use. The responsibility of employed to employer and the fear of loss of pay or job are not the prime forces which keep them at work. More important are the conventions about industry, the reproof which laziness is likely to draw from a man's fellows,[2] and the stimulus given by work in company with songs and jokes which lighten drudgery and give it some tinge of recreation. It is significant, too, that for really heavy work such as dragging a log or a canoe many peoples have adopted rhythm as a guide and lightener of the labour. Not only does a working song like a sailor's shanty give the time for pulling together, but it also distracts the mind from the dullness of the task.

Another common feature of work in a non-industrial society is the close association between technical and ritual activities. In theory it is easy to draw the distinction between these, but in practice the acts which produce the result desired are interwoven with a set of performances directed towards the promotion of fertility; the control of what we would regard as the incalculable factors of chance and of Nature; and the intervention of ancestors or gods on behalf of human effort. It has been pointed out by Malinowski and other anthropologists that this ritual is not a mere drag upon the economic activity but plays an important part in integrating the efforts of the workers and in giving confidence in the face of what might be the inhibiting fear of the unknown. On the other hand, these ritual performances, and the beliefs which they express, do appear at times to operate against the efficiency of the economic process, by leading to the retention of traditional technique of a less efficient kind than might be discovered by freer experimental methods. They also absorb time which might be devoted to the increase of wealth in other directions. Still, it must be remembered that considering the attitude to time already mentioned, the discarding of magical or ritual accompaniments to work might not increase the efficiency of the productive process. It has been shown that the abandonment of the ritual of agriculture in communities under European influence, such as the Maori, has reacted unfavourably upon the quality of the work performed.

It is difficult to speak of capital in a non-industrial economy in a way which makes it comparable with the idea in our own society. People outside an industrial market system do devote certain types of goods to facilitating production, and from time to time accumulate them in advance for this specific purpose. Thus, before starting to have a canoe built, a Tikopia man may plant extra areas of food and see that the woman of his household get in stock a quantity of barkcloth and pandanus mats additional to normal requirements. But this capital is fluid in its nature, and the objects so used can be at once

76

turned to a variety of other purposes if the need arises. Should a person die in the man's family before he starts his canoe-building, or even during the process of his work, the goods accumulated will be turned into material for a series of funeral exchanges. The mobility of 'capital' is high in such societies; diversion to other uses without loss is usually possible. The investment of capital with definite idea of getting a return from it in the form of interest is, however, not at all common. Where goods are contributed by others to assist a man in productive enterprise, these are usually given either in accordance with kinship obligations or as part of a general scheme of reciprocal arrangements, and are transferred back again with no additional increment.

This last point brings up the problem of exchange. Prior to contact with Europeans many pre-industrial communities had no objects which could properly be called 'money', and, therefore, no price system. Such communities are commonly spoken of as practising barter. But as an equivalent of buying and selling on a non-price level, barter implies the idea of haggling, in the attempt by each party to secure the highest return for what he hands over. Now this is by no means always the case in a non-industrial transaction. Not only are customary rates of exchange common, but the traditional factor which guides these rates is not mere inertia, but a complex set of ideas about liberality, respect for the personality of the other party, and for the act of exchange as one of social linkage wider than the purely material transaction. This reaches its highest form in what has been termed the 'gift exchange'. Here a recognised rate is observed, and the principle of reciprocity operates, but the form of the transaction is that of a gift and a counter-gift – between gentlemen, so to speak, avoiding the notion of haggling as being derogatory to the social position of both. At times, in fact, the recipient of the first gift deliberately makes his return gift higher in value in order to maintain his social standing. Another feature of such transactions is the existence of what may be termed 'spheres of exchange'. There are various groups of goods and services, and exchange of one item can only take place with another item in the same group. In south-eastern New Guinea, for instance, a very important series of exchanges takes place between the possessors of shell arm-rings and of necklaces of shell discs, while other important exchanges are of fish for vegetables. But

77

the food items can only be exchanged against each other, and so also the shell valuables. It would be unthinkable for a man who wished a shell valuable to offer in return yams or fish or other property not of a shell kind. There is no free market, no final measure of the value of individual things, and no common medium whereby every type of goods and services can be translated into terms of every other. A 'primitive' economy thus presents a strong contrast to our money economy.

A non-market distributive system, therefore, does not consist of finding exact equivalents for the services rendered by the different factors of production. It tends rather to follow the conception of reward for the social advantages conferred by participation in production, instead of a quantitative return for the material advantage obtained. The categories of wages, interest, and profit cannot easily be isolated in such a system. Moreover, the needs of the component members of the society are taken directly into account, so that the system is governed by principles of welfare and justice which vary according to the particular community. But such communities cannot be classed as communistic in any exact sense of the term. There are concepts of property-holding, and the means of production are held in ownership by individuals as well as by groups. Frequently these individual property rights are of a very complicated character. They may be based upon ties with father's and with mother's kin, and involve the rights of women in the family goods, and of chiefs in the goods of the people of their clan. At the same time the theory of corporate responsibility is usually well developed, restraining individuals from the exploitation of their fellows by moral codes of considerable force.

Some of the complexities of economic systems studied primarily by anthropologists should now be obvious. It is impossible to give detailed consideration to every point. But one cardinal feature of many an economic system of tribal peoples has been clearly the absence of money, of a price mechanism, and in many cases of a formal market. We may take this as symptomatic of the economy as a whole. Because of this situation it may be thought that the economy operates without clear principle, that transactions take place either in a kind of individual anarchy, or, as Marshall put it, 'by hereditary habit'.

In our own economic system money gives an almost universal

78

measure of values, a convenient medium of exchange through which we can buy or sell almost anything, and also a standard by which payments at one time can be expressed as commitments for the future. In a wider sense it allows for the measurement of services against things, and promotes the flow of the economic process. In a society without money we might expect all this to be absent, yet the economic process goes on. There is a recognition of services, and payment is made for them; there are means of absorbing people into the productive process, and values are expressed in quantitative terms, measured by traditional standards.

Let us examine, to begin with, a situation of simple distribution such as occurs when an animal is killed in a hunt. Do the hunters fall on the carcass and cut it to pieces, the largest piece to the strongest man? This is hardly ever the case. The beast is normally divided according to recognised principles. Since the killing of an animal is usually a co-operative activity one might expect to find it portioned out according to the amount of work done by each hunter to obtain it. To some extent this principle is followed, but other people have their rights as well. Traditionally, in many parts of Australia each person in the camp gets a share depending upon his or her relation to the hunters. The worst parts may even be kept by the hunters themselves. In former times, at Alice Springs, when a kangaroo was killed the hunter had to give the left hind leg to his brother, the tail to his father's brother's son, the loins and fat to his father-in-law, the ribs to his mother-in-law, the forelegs to his father's younger sister, the head to his wife, and he kept for himself the entrails and the blood. In different areas the portions assigned to such kinsfolk differ. When grumbles and fights occur, as they often do, it is not because the basic principles of distribution are questioned, but because it is thought they are not being properly followed. Though the hunter, his wife, and children seem to fare badly, this inequality is corrected by their getting in their turn better portions from kills by other people. The result is a criss-cross set of exchanges always in progress. The net result in the long run is substantially the same to each person, but through this system the principles of kinship obligation and the morality of sharing foods have been emphasised.

We see from this that though the principle that a person should get a reward for his labour it not ignored, this principle is caught up into

79

a wider set of codes which recognise that kinship ties, positions, or privilege, and ritual ideas should be supported on an economic basis. As compared with western capitalist society, Asian, Oceanian and other pre-capitalist societies often make direct allowance for the dependants upon producers as well as for the immediate producers themselves.

These same principles come out in an even more striking way in the feasts which are such an important part of much tribal life. The people who produce the food, or who own it, deliberately often hand over the best portions to others.

A feast may be the means of repaying the labour of others; of setting the seal on an important event, such as initiation or marriage; or of cementing an alliance between groups. Prestige is usually gained by the giver of the feast, but where personal credit and renown are linked most closely with the expenditure of wealth the giving of a feast is a step upon the ladder of social status. In the Banks Islands and other parts of Melanesia such feasts are part of the ceremonial of attaining the various ranks of the men's society, which is an important feature of local life. In Polynesia these graded feasts do not normally occur, but in Tikopia a chief is expected to mark the progress of his reign by a feast every decade or so. The 'feasts of merit' of the Nagas of Assam are not so much assertion against social com-

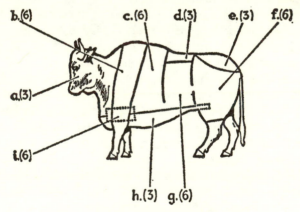

Fig. 2 – Division of meat at a Chin feast
(After H. N. C. Stevenson)

80

petitors as means of gaining certain recognised ranks in the society.

Let us take as an example the feast of *Khuang tsawi*, the greatest feast of all among the Zahau Chins of Burma, which has been described by H. N. C. Stevenson. A most important feature of this feast is the killing and division of the meat of three of the curious kind of cattle known as *mithan*. The flesh of the animal is not cut up at random, but is divided into a series of recognised joints, each of which has its own name. Moreover, each type of joint must be handed over to a particular class of people. Fig. 2 shows the way in which the animal is cut up. The following table gives the distribution of the various joints. It will be remembered that three of the animals are killed; the numbers given after each joint indicate the total number of pieces available for distribution:

Joint	Number	Recipients
a	3	Divided between father, brother, and father's brothers' sons. After the meat is taken off the skulls are returned to the feast-giver, who hangs them up in front of his house as a sign of his wealth.
b	6	1 to feast-giver; 1 to a scape-goat (an idiot on whom ill-luck should fall); 1 to supplier of bamboo for a chair for the feast-giver's wife; 1 to an assistant; 2 to former feast-givers.
c	6	6 to former feast-givers.
d	3	1 to headman; 2 to bond-friends.
e	3	Divided between father, brother, and father's brothers' sons.
f	6	3 to former feast-givers; 3 to sisters or close female cousins.
g	6	6 to assistants.
h	3	3 to 'working-sisters' that is, to female relatives, not very closely related, who help in the work.
i	6	1 to headman; 2 to former feast-givers; others not mentioned.

In addition to this, three portions of flesh beneath the breast-bone are given to the blacksmith; the entrails to a wife's brother and a mother's brother of the feast-giver; blood in sausages warmed with slivers of meat and some small portions of flesh to widows and the destitute.

In this complicated scheme of distribution we see that three main sets of people receive meat. One set are kinsfolk of the feast-giver; another set are people who have performed services for him (including his two friends the blacksmith and the headman); and the third set are the givers of former feasts. The deference shown to this last

81

set of people is a token of how in this community a man builds up his social position by a free use of his wealth. When he himself has given a feast, then he gets more meat and better beer at future feasts given by other people; he gets a higher bride price for his daughters when they marry; he becomes eligible for membership of the village council; and, if he goes on with his feast-giving, he earns the right to make windows in his house, and to build a little summer-house on the platform of his courtyard. And finally, by the *Khuang tsawi* feast he becomes eligible to enter at his death the highest heaven of the Chin people. Among the Chin, as among many other people, it is more blessed to give than to receive, but only because the act of giving entitles one to receive more at a future date.

This ceremonial division of animals at a feast is a common feature. Peter Buck has described the division of pigs, bonito, and shark in Samoa. A pig is divided up into ten portions, each of which has its name, and is appropriate to people of a certain rank or status. So important is the ceremonial division of a Samoan pig that the quality of the food becomes a secondary affair. If the pig is too well cooked, then the flesh is likely to tear when cut, and the exact boundaries of the ceremonial division cannot be kept. Then the hosts are ashamed and the people who get the joints are critical. The result is that the pig is often served nearly raw. Not that the Samoans like raw pork to eat. The guest is not expected to consume his share immediately; he satisfies himself with the fish and vegetables which go with it. The important thing is not for him to eat the pork, but for him to have been *given* it. So highly have the Samoans developed their system of etiquette and of social precedence that our rules of behaviour, even on formal occasions, seem crude and unorganised beside theirs.

We may now consider how inequalities in possession of resources between different people are met, in the absence of a monetary commercial system. The absence of money does not mean that there is no exchange. Even among very isolated peoples there is usually some contact with other tribes and some exchange of things between them. Sometimes there are regular markets, as used to occur in Malaita in the Solomon Islands, and still do in many parts of Africa; often exchange takes place as the result of expeditions sent out for the purpose.

Trading expeditions of a dramatic kind have been recorded among

82

the tribes of the New Guinea coast. The *hiri* of the Motu, described by Seligman and Barton, and the *kula* of the Trobriand Islands, described by Malinowski, have in fact, become classical accounts of seafaring among native people.

The Motu, who live in a dry belt of Papua, and whose women are potters, set out each year at the end of the south-east trade wind with a cargo of pots on a 200-mile voyage. They return six months later, before the end of the north-west monsoon, with a raft of new dug-out canoes and tons of sago in their holds. Each voyage is an adventure with risk, so it is not surprising to find that taboos are laid in plenty both on the sailors and on their wives at home, and that magic is performed to promote the sailing powers of the canoe and avert shipwreck. The Trobrianders, who participate in the famous *kula*, carry on two types of exchange, the one of useful articles such as pots, the other of necklaces of red shell and bracelets of white shell, which, though ornaments, are hardly ever worn. The necklaces are exchanged between partners in the various island groups through a circle of several hundred miles, and move in the direction of the hands of a clock. The arm-shells move likewise, but in the opposite direction, and are exchanged for the necklaces as they meet them. These exchanges are of a complicated kind, and take the form of reciprocal gifts, often months apart. They take place mostly by means of special expeditions in canoes, and like the canoes of the *hiri* those of the *kula* are built and sailed in the midst of a cloud of magic. This *kula* institution draws our attention to one feature of Oceanic exchange which is extremely important, namely, that this exchange often reaches its highest peak, not with objects of ordinary domestic use, but with things which may be of little or no practical use. They have their value, as it were, through their elevation in exchange, and not for any outside reason. In a sense the exchange itself is the thing of value, and not the object.

There are regions, however, where ceremonial exchange is carried on without regular expeditions. The opportunity for exchange is given by large inter-tribal gatherings for initiation or other ceremonials. Such is the case of the Mulluk Mulluk and Madngella of the Daly River in northern Australia, as described by W. E. H. Stanner. The system is termed *merbok*. A great variety of articles travel along the *merbok* paths. They include iron oxides, pipe-clay, hair belts, spears,

83

boomerangs, beeswax, pearl-shell ornaments, stone axes, and knives. Some of these articles are not actually used by certain of the tribes who exchange them; they merely pass the things on to their partners in the opposite direction. Many of these articles go immense distances; pearl-shell from the west coast has been found hundreds of miles inland, and a type of boomerang characteristic of tribes around Wave Hill has been seen among tribes of the Finniss and Daly rivers over 200 miles to the north.[3] Nowadays many European articles pass along the *merbok* paths in this way.

The *merbok* exchange, like those of New Guinea, is carried on between definite partners, all of whom in this case are kinsfolk of one kind or another. The transactions take place with little fuss. But they have a ceremonial side, since they do not serve merely utilitarian ends, and the possession of a partner is in itself a mark of social maturity. The transient possession of a store of objects, even though he himself does not use them, gives a man a satisfaction, especially when he can hand them on to others and receive a return. Moreover, the gift of an object is a mark of friendship, and serves to strengthen social bonds which are of value in other directions. But the position of a *merbok* partner is not always an easy one. He often has to decide whether, for instance, he will divert an object from one of his partners to meet a claim raised by marriage or the initiation of his sister's son. If he does so, then he will have to find an equivalent object soon or risk his partner's anger, detrimental gossip, possible attempt at sorcery, or even a challenge to fight. (Analogous problems of decision occur in the *kula*.)

Among many Oceanic peoples occasions of human rejoicing or sadness are treated as an opportunity for complicated exchanges of goods, and from their point of view the expression of the appropriate emotions would not be fully possible without such exchanges. Vast quantities of goods may then change hands. At one betrothel in Ontong Java in the Solomon Islands Hogbin records that 16,000 coconuts and ten large baskets of dried fish were given to the parents of the girl by the boy's father. This gift increased the respect in which the donor was generally held. But a few weeks later, when another man gave 17,000 coconuts as a betrothal present for his son, he was criticised as a vulgar boaster, and felt himself to be so unpopular that he retired to an island out of public view for some months. Frequently custom prescribes that the goods from the bridegroom's and the bride's family should be of different types. In Samoa, for instance, the relatives of the bridegroom gave the *oloa* of canoes, pigs, and other food, while the relatives of the bride presented in return the *tonga* of beautiful fine mats of native craft. When a marriage took place between Maori people of rank, heirlooms were exchanged and served future generations as a token of the union between the noble families. Such an heirloom as a valued neck ornament might be handed back to the original donors many years later at a death in their family. It was then described as *roimata*, 'tears', a description which indicates the imagery of the Maori. Sometimes such exchanges serve utilitarian purposes by providing the other party with goods not previously in their possession. More often the gain is not so much in terms of useful objects as in the social value of the exchange itself.

We have already stated that money is not a characteristic feature of many non-industrial economic systems. Yet the terms 'primitive currency' and 'primitive money' have been commonly used. They have been applied to a wide variety of objects of value: coconuts in the Nicobar Islands; cowrie shells, hoes, and spear-heads in Africa; pigs and strings of shell discs in the New Hebrides, the Solomon Islands, and New Guinea; shields in Guadalcanal; coils of red feathers in Santa Cruz; whales' teeth in Fiji; beeswax in Borneo; and glass jars in Burma. How far are these terms accurate? We have already described the function of money in conventional terms as giving a medium of exchange between other objects and a measure of their value. From this point of view some of the items mentioned seem to be fairly described. Coconuts in the Nicobar Islands, we learn, once had the functions of money. Thus, needles were exchanged at twelve coconuts per dozen, matches at twenty-four nuts per dozen boxes, and red cloth at 1,600 coconuts per piece. Moreover, though payment need not be made in nuts, they served as a measure of values. A racing canoe was bought for 35,000 coconuts. But this was simply a measure of its value. The payment was made in cloth, beads, and implements which themselves were valued in terms of nuts. The money of India, too, had its value in terms of Nicobar coconuts. A two-anna bit was worth sixteen nuts, a rupee, one hundred nuts. Since a two-anna bit was one-eighth of a rupee it seems as if the multiplication of the Nicobar people was at fault. But the two coins were used for ornament as well as for exchange, and a rupee as a single coin was less prized for personal adornment than eight of the two-anna pieces. Here, then, coins were not simply money, but objects depending for their value upon other considerations, and the real objective standard was provided by coconuts. In many parts of Africa cowrie shells appear to perform the same function of currency or money.

On the other hand, items such as feather coils, shields, mats, and whales' teeth do not seem to be properly classified as primitive money. They are important items of exchange, but their transfer does not facilitate the exchange of other things, and they do not serve as a standard to which the values of other things can be referred. Even pigs, which are exchanged very freely, and the possession of which is a measure of a man's wealth in many of the South Sea islands, can hardly be called money. In Malekula, for instance, pigs are treasured for their tusks, and quality is much more important than quantity. Sows are of no social importance and are regarded as food fit only for women and children. With boars the two upper canine teeth are knocked out while the animal is young, with the result that the lower teeth grow longer and longer, curving round till they pierce the lower jaw and sometimes even grow out again in more than a complete circle. There are many grades of value of these boars, the index being their tusk development. Each grade has its name and special function. For the higher grades special gong signals are sounded when at a feast the animal is presented or killed. All important ceremonies are bound up with pig-killing, and the borrowing, lending, and transfer of these animals. As many as a hundred or a hundred and fifty pigs may be distributed at one of these ceremonies. The social importance of these animals, their graded values, and the credit transactions that take place with them still do not entitle them to be termed money in the strict economic sense. But what is important to observe is that without a money system as ordinarily defined, these people manage an economic scheme of considerable complexity, have standards of value, and exchange freely large quantities of goods.

The classification of strings of shell discs which are used freely in the western Pacific is more difficult. Malinowski has shown the need for scepticism about the classing of an object as 'primitive money' unless it can be shown that the mechanism of exchange among a people requires the existence of an article to be used as a common medium of exchange and measure of value. He has rightly pointed out that the valued shell ornaments exchanged in the *kula* ring are never used in this way. They are condensed wealth, to which is attached a complex sentiment aroused by competitive desire and by the ritual use of these objects, but they are not money.

It does seem, though, that in the Solomon Islands and the Banks Islands strings of shell discs at times have played this rôle. In Buin, Thurnwald has described the use of fathoms of shell discs, one fathom being valued at a shilling. In olden times spears, arrows, bows, stone axe-blades, and clam shell arm-rings were sometimes traded for these shell strings; and until recently fishing nets, bags, painted hats, combs, bamboo cases for lime, native tobacco, and European products were freely bought and sold with them. There are no markets, but bargains were made between individuals at casual meetings. Pigs, too, which are very important as an index of a man's wealth and the chief item in feasts, are exchanged for these shell strings – from ten or twenty up to one hundred fathoms. Thurnwald speaks, in fact, of a 'pig standard of currency', since the value of the shell strings lies largely in their ability to be converted into pigs, which are in turn the fundamental element in a feast, which itself is the pivot on which the social and economic life turns.

Another interesting system has been recorded by Armstrong from Rossel Island, to the south-east of New Guinea. Here there are two types of shell discs, one called *dap* and the other *kö*. Of *dap* there are twenty-two classes, each with a name and comprising a number of single reddish triangular pieces of shell. In classes fifteen to twenty-two each coin has an individual name; there are eighty-one of them in all, and each is known individually to men with financial interests. *Kö* is a unit of ten discs of clam shell, and there are sixteen classes of it. The first is equivalent in name to the seventh class of *dap*, so that No. 16 *kö* equals No. 22 *dap* in name. There is no real equivalence of value between them; they are not exchanged for each other. In each of the two groups the value of an item in one class is proportionate to that of an item in a class below it, according to the amount of time taken before the latter must be repaid by the former. Thus, if a No. 7 *dap* is lent for a few days a No. 8 *dap* must be given in return for it; if for some weeks, then a No. 9 or 10 must be returned. These objects circulate a great deal. They are used to buy other articles, and are borrowed for the purpose, being repaid after some time by the appropriate piece that the borrower possesses. There are brokers, too, who lend these objects and get those of higher value in return.

But though these shell strings are very freely used, and the values of many other objects can be expressed in terms of them, they still do not appear to have that universal applicability which money has attained in our own society. Coins of the highest value have to be handled with much ceremonial. When one of No. 18 *dap* is handed over from one person to another both parties crouch down out of respect to it. Nos. 19 to 22 *dap* are so sacred that they are not supposed to see the light of day, and are always kept enclosed. They are owned only by chiefs, and function only as security for loans. Of No. 22 there are only seven coins, inherited in the male line, and the chiefs who own them are apparently the most important in the island. Again, *dap* and *kö* cannot be expressed in terms of each other as our coins of different metal can. *Kö* is to some extent women's money. And items of higher value are individualised and have personal names. Armstrong maintains that these shell articles are really money in the strict sense. Not only do they serve as a medium of exchange and as a standard of value, he says, but they are not desired for their utility for other purposes, even for ornament or display. But it is not clear that his classification can be accepted, and recent field study has indicated that the system is more complex and less finely calculated in time-span terms than Armstrong realised. In their use for special ritual purposes, those shell discs of the highest value at least seem to be objects of wealth in themselves, and something more than money.

In a community without true money, how are the values of goods determined, and indeed have they any value at all? The answer to this question depends upon the meaning we attach to 'value'. We can perhaps agree that things have no intrinsic value in themselves apart from their relation to people and people's wants. If, in the first place, we think that value is 'price', then values obviously cannot be measured in a community without money. If, then, by value we mean the cost of making a thing, we cannot measure non-monetary values in this sense either, because relative costs can be measured only in the vaguest way. The labour-cost theory of value, which has sometimes been put forward, has very little meaning because of the absence of any exact calculation of time spent, or of any final distinction between work and recreation, and because the relation between skilled and unskilled labour is not clearly defined. In any case, cost alone cannot be a clue to non-monetary values because the reasons which lead people to want things are often independent of the difficulties of producing them. By value in our buying-and-selling society we usually mean exchange-value. But in many pre-industrial societies, as we have seen, there is no attempt to exchange each kind of object against another, and no medium which can express their comparative worth for exchange purposes. A purist might then argue that *economic values* do not exist in many pre-industrial societies. Every society does, however, appear to have some rating of the worth of different kinds of things outside the sphere of their immediate practical use. Some kind of comparison between them usually takes place as by the limited exchanges of trade or ceremony which we have already described. And the preferences shown seem to have a more general application than those of simple individual taste. Thus an Australian aborigine may be expected always to prefer a shell pubic pendant to a hair belt; a Polynesian, a canoe to a piece of plain barkcloth; an African, a cow to a goat. There is, then, some sort of scale of comparative utilities or wants, though, especially in the cultures of simplest technical development, the scale is not finely adjusted, and there is no exact expression of the worth of one object in terms of another.

NOTES

1 *Principles of Economics*, p. 243 (8th edn, 1922).
2 The Maori people formerly used proverbs a great deal to spur on laggards or to praise the industrious man.
3 For the benefit of those who think that every Australian aborigine uses a boomerang, it may be noted that boomerangs are one type of object which are taken in exchange by the Daly River tribes, but are not used by them.

CHAPTER FOUR

Some Principles of Social Structure

LIFE in a community means organisation of the interests of individuals, regulation of their behaviour towards one another, and grouping them together for common action. The relationships thus created between them can be seen to have some kind of plan or system, which may be called the *social structure*. The way in which the relationships actually work, affecting the lives of individuals and the nature of the society, may be called their *social functions*. Social structure and social function may be compared with the anatomy and physiology of a biological organism, though the studies of either cannot be kept separate. The analogy is not an exact one, since the individual people who compose a human society are much more mobile and more complex than the cell units of a biological organism. But the comparison may be useful.[1]

The social structure of a community includes the different types of groups which the people form and the institutions in which they take part. When we speak of an institution we mean certain sets of relationships arising from the activities of groups of people with a social end to accomplish. The social structure, both as regards groups and institutions, can be seen to be based upon definite principles. Sex, age, locality, and kinship are among the most fundamental of these in all human societies. We shall see better how these principles of grouping work by examining non-industrial societies with their smaller size and simpler organisation rather than the larger and complicated industrial societies.

Consider first sex division. Men and women are marked off from each other by differences in dress, name, and ordinary habits. This division is seen also in the economic sphere. In non-industrial communities hunting, fishing, woodwork, metal-work, and the tending of cattle are more often the tasks of men while looking after the home and children, agriculture, and the making of clothing are usually the work of women. Where agriculture is shared, the men often have to do the heavier work of breaking up the soil, while the women come in later to tend and weed the plants. In a fishing community the women may go out with small hand nets and scoop up what fish and crabs they can get on the reef, while the men use a greater variety of apparatus, and in particular go out in canoes off the shore for deep-sea fishing. No man would use a woman's handnet – although he is the maker of it – and no woman is allowed to fish from a canoe.

The sex division goes deeper than an agreement upon clothes or a sharing out of tasks. Not only questions of convenience and habit, but also ideas of what should be done, complicate the position. If members of one sex do not obey the custom, and, in particular, try to adopt the habits of the other sex, then strong feelings of ridicule, anger, and even religious emotion may be aroused. In more self-conscious and intellectualised communities such ideas are often based upon notions of psychological differences between men and women. Many societies do not try and rationalise sex attitudes in this way, but are content to base the differences upon tradition. Sometimes these traditional rules impose actual disabilities upon women, but frequently this is more apparent than real. Whatever be her theoretical social position, in practice a woman exerts a very considerable influence. For instance, in a society where women are supposed to be ignorant of the sacred lore I have heard a wife prompt her husband when such matters were discussed. Again, where women are excluded from certain aspects of the social organisation, as in the men's secret societies of the New Hebrides and of West Africa, they frequently have compensation in the possession of secret organisations of their own, from which men in turn are kept out.

These social differences between the sexes which occur in every type of human society may ultimately be related to the biological position of woman as the child-bearer. Her specialisation of bodily function may be associated with certain psychological differences, but of this we have less evidence. But, like many other systems of human rules, those concerned with the behaviour of the sexes have grown away from their original foundation. In a sense social codes now create sex difference almost more than they express it. This can be seen from the fact that the behaviour attributed to women in one society may be exactly the reverse in another society. Take the length

91

of the hair. In England her hair is a woman's crowning glory, and she wears it rather longer than that of her husband or brother. But in Tikopia it is the custom for women to crop their hair close to the head, and for men, especially young men, to wear it long down their backs. This custom is not a matter of simple taste or habit. It is linked with dancing and mourning. A favourite dance is that called the 'canoe bow', in which the head is waved from side to side so that the masses of hair toss like the spray as the craft is forced through the waves. The young men are very proud of their long tresses.[2] When a relative dies, one of their greatest sacrifices in mourning is to cut their hair. Dancing is prohibited during mourning, so that social restraint and short hair go together. Thus the differences of custom between the sexes, though arbitrary in their origin, are intelligible in terms of the particular codes of the society where they are found.

Some kind of division and stratification of peoples always exists on a basis of age. In Polynesia respect for elders is basic in the social life. Such a proverb as 'have respect to me, a setting sun, a fallen tree, stricken by many waters', when uttered by an old Maori man, has been often sufficient to get him much more favourable treatment than he otherwise might have got. Respect for the aged is well known as a feature of Chinese society. In aboriginal Australia the age principle comes out in the control which older men exercise over boys and younger men, in the ordeals they inflict upon them in initiation cere- monies, and the general guidance which they give through their superior knowledge. Here the system of naming kinsfolk itself empha- sises the age differentiation by opposing very strongly people of alternate generations, such as father and son. The importance of the linkage of age and experience is seen elsewhere in the frequent exis- tence of councils of elders, who act either as advisers to chiefs or as the final authority in a tribe.

In many societies, as in our own western society, the grouping of people on an age principle is fairly fluid. But in some non-industrial communities a system of what are generally called age-grades is an integral part of the social structure. This has been particularly so among some Plains Indians of North America and some East African tribes. The Nandi of Kenya, described by Hollis, may be taken as an illustration. When Hollis wrote, in 1909, there were seven grades of Nandi males, each made up of people whose ages were within about ten years of one another. The great event among the East African tribes which ushers people into this system is the initiation festival. This takes place, with the Nandi, every seven or eight years, upon a group of boys and adolescents aged from about ten to twenty, but mostly from fifteen to nineteen. Before initiation a boy belongs to the first grade, which does not count in the same way as the others. At initiation the lads are circumcised, they are beaten with stinging nettles, and hornets are dropped on their backs to try their courage further. Later they are instructed in their duty as warriors. Every one initiated at the same septennial ceremony belongs to the same grade, or 'set' as it is perhaps better called, which has a definite name, emblems, and ornaments. A man then goes through life together with his comrades, doing the same tasks as they do, having the same social status, and sharing the same privileges. After marriage, a man is expected to give an age-mate hospitality, and even to let him sleep with his wife – a service he does not give outside the 'age-set'. Each age-set is still further divided into three sections called 'fires', also on an age basis, and these remain aloof from one another in their camping arrangements. The junior sets are the warriors; these later marry, and hand over their task while they carry on the ordinary business of the tribe, including procreation; later, they become elders, responsible for advice and the maintenance of the law. As warriors the young men are allowed regular sex relationships but may not marry or have children. Every seven or eight years – about four years after the initiation rite – the Nandi used to hold a definite ceremony of 'handing over the country' by the senior men to the junior set of warriors. A white bullock was sacrificed; the age-set retiring from active warrior life took off their garments and put on those of elders, and the warriors of the set now in power were solemnly told that the welfare of the land of their fathers and of the people was put in their hands.

The age-grades are not really absolute divisions; there is always some overlap, and it is possible for wealthy orphans or for the sons of old men to be initiated earlier than usual. Some lads, on the other hand, may have to wait a long time. The common term 'age-grade' may be misleading. The sets of men do not move up from one grade into another as boys move through forms at school. They take their grade with them in a sense, name, insignia, and all; they change only the rôle which they have to play.

What the age-grade system does as a whole in these tribes is to mark off in a broad formal way the generation levels, and institutionalise certain important social groupings and codes of behaviour by reference to advancing years. It provides for respect to seniors and training of juniors; it organises sex relations and the time of marriage; sets up a specific grouping for warfare; and provides for a regular transfer of the responsibility for external security.

Societies graded by age among the Plains Indians are confined to five tribes – the Hidatsa, Mandan, Arapaho, Gros Ventre, and Blackfoot. Among the Hidatsa there used to be about a dozen of these societies. They bore names such as Stone Hammer, Little Dogs, Kit Foxes, Half-Shaved Heads, and Black Mouths. Each had its own emblem and regalia, special dances, and peculiar functions and privileges. The Stone Hammers had licence to steal food after public announcements; the Black Mouths acted as police. Most of the societies incited their members to distinguish themselves in war. Membership, or rather ownership of each society, was obtained by a group of age-mates purchasing the rights in it collectively from an older group. Apparently elders never bought societies from younger people. Buyers and sellers were regarded as standing ceremonially in the relation of 'sons' and 'fathers' respectively.

There was a definite progression through these societies with advancing age. The feeling of moving with the age-group was strong. It was felt that a man should belong to the same age-society as his age-mate. But, unlike the sets of the East African tribes, there was no association of a definite society with a definite age. The basis of membership of the society was purchase, and not age as such. This is shown by the fact that if the members of a society wanted too high a price to hand it over, or their juniors were unwilling to buy it, then it might remain in their ownership for years, and they might even acquire another as well. One can talk of age-grades here, then, only in terms of a general trend or sequence. The ladder is of a telescopic and not of a rigid type. Where the age principle enters in is to give a useful basis for getting people together for an act of collective purchase and enjoyment of special ornaments and privileges.

In parts of Melanesia there are societies or clubs which have a complicated system of grades and ranks, and which seem superficially to resemble those we have just discussed. But their relationship with age groupings is only incidental, and they are basically an expression of rank and privilege in terms of wealth.

Grouping of people on the basis of their common residence is extremely important. In the smaller unit, such as household, nomadic camp, or settled village, or hamlet, the very fact of living in close touch forces people to co-operate in work and in play, and to adopt some unity of attitude on many of their common problems. But though the tie of locality can be strong in creating and maintaining human groups, it is usually reinforced by other principles such as those of kinship.

In many non-industrial societies a unit which relies a great deal on local associations is the tribe. This is sometimes spoken of as a group of people of a cultural order, that is, normally occupying a common territory, speaking a common language, and in particular having in common a set of traditions and institutions and responding to the same government. It is sometimes difficult, however, to decide whether two groups of people historically related should be regarded as sub-tribes or as separate tribes.

The tie of common residence and common ownership of lands is an important one in pre-industrial hunting and agricultural communities. Local patriotism is often well developed. It has been found difficult to get Western Australian shepherds to herd sheep off the territory of their own local group. Travellers have frequently expressed the desire when nearing death to be buried on their own land. And several times in Maori history the statement of a chief, 'let me die on my land', has been sufficient to rally his warriors and beat back the enemy.

Another most important principle of social grouping is that of kinship. This may be defined as the bonds of blood and marriage, or more precisely the system of social ties based on the recognition of genealogical relationships, that is, those resulting from legalised sex union and the procreation of children. The idea that kinship is an important tie finds expression in a number of ways. Many types of social group have this as their cementing factor. Other groups of an economic or a political kind often rely on kinship to a large extent for their effectiveness, and from kinship relations spring moral values

95

of the most intense character. Mother-love, a kinship sentiment, is the most obvious example of this.

The most fundamental way in which kinship is effective in social life is through the family. In common speech the word 'family' may mean several different things, but when the sociologist or anthropologist uses the term, he means the small group of parents and children. The family is regarded as being incomplete unless the three elements – father, mother, and child – are present. The 'eternal triangle' of the stage and screen is of two men and one woman (nowadays sometimes two women and one man) in a state of conflicting passions. The real 'eternal triangle' as the anthropologist sees it is the child with its father and its mother, united by common sentiment – the elementary family.

In every human society which has been examined scientifically the family organisation has been found as a basic unit, even among pygmies and other peoples of simple technology. Sometimes it has been veiled by customs which have led observers to infer states of promiscuity, group marriage, and communal rearing of children. Such conditions have been stated to exist among the tribes of aboriginal Australia. But investigations by Malinowski, Radcliffe-Brown, and later workers have shown that real family life as we understand it underlies even the wildest aberrations of sexual life.[3]

The reasons for this universality of the family as a human group are easy to see. They lie in biological and social needs, first of the pregnant woman and then of the mother and child. But this satisfaction of biological requirements does not exhaust the situation. Since the young of Man requires a very much longer time to attain maturity than that of other animals the process of education is also prolonged. One of the most valuable functions of parenthood lies in handing on to the child by example, as well as by instruction, a very great deal of the cultural heritage of the group to which the parents belong. So far no substitute, whether communal nursery or enlightened school system, has been able to replace the family entirely in this respect. More and more psychology recognises the importance of the formative influences brought to bear on the child in its early infancy. Implicitly, human societies everywhere have anticipated these findings by the fundamental rôle they assign to the family. Put another way, it may be said that the societies themselves have, in fact, been founded on the family organisation.

A distinction must be drawn between the basic structure of the family and its external form. The same components of father, mother, and children, closely united by ties of mutual help and sentiment, exist in all societies. But the setting is often very different. The form of marriage, the distribution of authority in the household, the systems of occupation and of residence, the transmission of descent, the conception of parenthood, the prevalence of customs such as adoption and divorce, and the presence of larger kinship groups such as the clan, all tend to provide different moulds in which the fluid elements of family life must set.

Consider first the form of marriage. We in Europe are so used to monogamy as the type of marriage laid down by law and by Christian morality that we often fail to realise that over other large areas of the world different types of marriage exist, not as deviations from a monogamous ideal, but as ideals in themselves.

Polygamy – in the form of marriage with more than one wife – is very common in the Muslim countries, in China, in many parts of pagan Africa, and in Oceania. It is frequently, but by no means always, practised by wealthy men rather than poor men. Our aversion to polygamy is largely founded on the idea that a permanent sex relation between a man and more than one woman is repugnant. If such a relation exists in our own society it is normally kept secret. But to think of polygamy primarily in terms of sex relations is to misunderstand it.

The kind of reasons which lie at the base of it in an African society may be seen from a consideration of the custom among two tribes of Tanzania, the Nyakyusa, studied by Godfrey Wilson, and the Hehe, studied by Gordon Brown, in each of which polygamy was widespread. Among the Nyakyusa most polygamists were men of forty-five or over. From the tax registers in 1936, of 3,000 men in one area 34 per cent were found to be bachelors, 37 per cent monogamists, and 29 per cent polygamists. In a sample section of the Hehe, comprising over 4,000 taxpaying men, there were 25 per cent bachelors, 46 per cent monogamists, and 28 per cent polygamists. Among the Hehe, for every 100 married men there were, on the average, 153

97

married women; this was due to an actual excess of women over men, and to the earlier marriage of the women. Traditionally in both tribes polygamy is an ideal state which costs something to reach, but is regarded as well worth the trouble. The reasons recognised for it by the people include first, sexual satisfaction. This is not mere lust, but the satisfaction of what may be regarded as normal appetite, since there are taboos on intercourse with the mother of a child for some months after its birth. And among the Nyakyusa, the mother should not become pregnant again till the child has been weaned, which does not happen for two or three years, during which time the father is expected to have only restricted intercourse with his wife. Hence he takes other wives if he can. But the sex factor is only one single element, and not always the most important. Plurality of wives increases the probability of offspring, desired by both men and women. Again, there are economic reasons. A man's supply of labour is increased by his marrying additional wives. In a society where there is no hired labour, this is an important consideration. Among the Hehe if a man's wives are numerous enough he can escape the drudgery of agriculture. Linked with the greater productive powers thus afforded are the increase in wealth and prestige of the polygamist. He is able to give hospitality more freely, he gains in social esteem. Moreover, among both tribes, the father of a girl receives cattle from her husband at marriage, so that with polygamy his chances of increasing his herd are greater than with monogamy.

But in a polygamous marriage the man does not have all the benefits. If there is a surplus of women over men, as with the Hehe, they are absorbed, and not left in the kind of condition in which so many women found themselves in Britain after World War I. That polygamy is a condition approved by many women is seen from the fact that they normally enter it as free agents. It is extremely common for a Nyakyusa man to take as his second or third wife the sister, half-sister, or brother's daughter of his first wife (a custom known as the sororate). By so doing he pays a great compliment to this wife and her family; it shows he is satisfied with them. But the sister or cousin will not come to him unless she approves of him, and her consent likewise compliments him. Not uncommonly, in some non-industrial societies a wife will request her husband to take another wife, to lighten the work of the household.

What about family conditions in a polygamous marriage? Although the presence of other wives and children does give an enlarged family circle, the relation of the children and their mother in each case to their father still has an individuality and intimacy of its own. There is not a general pooling of children between the wives, but each suckles and tends her own, and has certain legal rights over them. The husband is, as it were, the single apex of a number of triangles at the base of each of which is a separate group of a wife and her children. One may speak of a polygamous family as a number of individual families, with a father in common. Frequently, especially in Africa, the wives have separate huts, and are visited by the husband in turn. Among the Hehe the father has responsibilities to each of his children, whether he is a polygamist or not: he is the head of the family and protector of all his children even after his daughter's marriage; he has an economic obligation to assist his son in finding the cattle needed for his marriage, and to refund his daughter's bride-cattle if she is divorced; he has to pass on to his children his clan-name and property when he dies. Each mother has rights and duties to her children by him. She must look after them; she has the right of visiting any children claimed by her husband if they should separate, and of keeping small children herself; she has to give her consent to her daughter's marriage, and receives one third of the cattle paid over by her daughter's husband. On the other hand, she has the duty of contributing one-third of the cattle which her son must pay for his bride – though this is often done for her by her brother.

Polyandry – marriage to more than one husband – is much less common than polygyny – marriage to more than one wife. But where it occurs the same reality of family life can be seen. Traditionally, when a Toda woman of the Nilgiri Hills, in south India, marries a man, it is understood that she becomes the wife of his brothers at the same time. When she becomes pregnant the eldest brother presents her with an imitation bow-and-arrow as a token of paternity of the child. All the brothers are said to be equally regarded as the fathers of the child. But if one of them leaves and sets up a house of his own, then it appears that he loses his right to the paternity. Moreover, in a few cases the husbands are not brothers. Here it is arranged beforehand which husband shall carry out the ceremony. He is the father of the child for all social purposes. All succeeding children belong to

99

him too, no matter who may be, or may be thought to be, the biological father, until another husband performs the same ceremony, when the next and following children belong to him. The net effect is that of several individual families with a wife and mother in common. So much does the fatherhood of the child depend on this ceremony that even a dead man may have children if no man has given the woman the bow-and-arrow in the meantime.

This last example raises the problem of the idea of parenthood held by different peoples. The physical tie of child with its mother is an obvious thing – it has clearly been born from her body. The ideas about the biological nature of this tie vary, however. Some peoples, for instance, are not clear about what part the woman plays in the conception of the child which appears in her womb, and when pregnancy really begins. Social motherhood again, involving the control of the child, may be different from physical motherhood. In some societies a child owes obedience first to its father's senior wife, and then to its own mother. The separation between the biological and the social ideas of parenthood is even clearer in the case of fatherhood. In Europe we regard the man who is responsible for the procreation of the child as its 'father' for social purposes – except where it has been adopted. But in some societies this is not so. The Todas, for example, by the bow-and-arrow ceremony lay all the emphasis on social fatherhood, and are content to let the biological aspect of paternity drop into the background. So also with many African peoples. The father of a child, from the social point of view, that is, from the point of authority, responsibility for its education, paying or receiving marriage gifts for it, and transmitting property to it – is the man who is married to the child's mother, or in some cases, who has paid cattle to secure these social rights. He is not necessarily the man who has actually begotten the child.

The most extreme example of the divorce of the idea of biological fatherhood from that of social fatherhood is seen with some Australian aborigines, and with the Trobrianders of New Guinea. The Trobrianders are in the position not simply of being ignorant as to what man is responsible for begetting a child, but of actually denying that a man has anything to do with begetting children at all. According to them sexual intercourse exists only for pleasure, and children are conceived by women because their ancestral spirits give them spirit

100

babies. All that a man can do is to 'open the way' through which a child may ultimately emerge, and even here he is not in theory necessary.[4] These views, surprising as they may seem, have been very fully documented by Malinowski, and verified later by Fortune and by Leo Austen. There is still argument among anthropologists as to exactly what literal and what symbolic meaning the Trobrianders have attached to such statements. But this emphatic denial by the Trobrianders of physical paternity can be closely linked with the strong emphasis they place upon matrilineal descent and inheritance. We might think to find, then, in this society sets of incomplete families – mothers and their children, but lacking the fathers we regard as essential for the children's welfare. But the Trobrianders, while hotly denying biological fatherhood, recognise social fatherhood as very important. A woman's husband is verbally a 'stranger', to use the local term, to his wife's children. But, in fact, he is their nurse, their protector, and their confidant; he takes a great part in their education, and hands over to them all kinds of gifts, even at the expense of his sisters' children, who are his legal heirs. According to the people themselves, it is a bad thing for an unmarried woman to bear a child, since it will not have a man 'to take it in his arms'.

In modern society the ties of kinship are less important for large-scale relationships than those of an economic or political kind. In non-industrial societies, however, kinship is often extremely important. Within the society kinship gives a basis for economic co-operation, for political unity, and for ritual assemblage; much of the code of etiquette of groups deals with the behaviour expected between kinsfolk. In societies such as the Australian aborigines, ties of kinship known to be traceable between groups of peoples a couple of hundred miles apart help visitors to receive hospitality, assure them of safety, and assist in trade. In a large-scale peasant community of coastal Malaysia I found people with only a few dozen kin, but in Tikopia, when the island had a population of 1,300 the people formed one group of relatives: I could find no two people who could not trace their kinship to each other.

For any group life to be successful there must be provision for its continuity – as people are born they must be incorporated into it upon some principle, and as people die the things that they possess must also be handed on according to rule. The way in which a person

101

acquires membership of a kinship group is termed *descent*. The way in which he acquires rank and privileges is termed *succession*, and the way in which he acquires material property after the death of its former owner is termed *inheritance*. The acquisition of such things, whether group membership, social status, or property, may take place through one parent or both. When it occurs through one parent only, on one side of the family, the principle is called *unilateral*; when through the two parents, on both sides of the family, it is called *bilateral*. These principles are usually consistent, generation after generation. But in some cases, while both sides of the family may be eligible for such transmission, because of residence or other reason only one is normally used, though there may be a shift from one side of the family to the other in successive generations. The principle here is one I have termed *ambilateral*. Kinship in general is bilateral, that is, the relationship as a whole normally involves ties through father (*patrilateral*) and through mother (*matrilateral*). Where continuity of group interests and transmission of rights through a line of ancestors is concerned, the terms *unilineal* and *bilineal* are used. Where the line of father's kin alone is followed, the system is *patrilineal*; where that of mother's kin, it is *matrilineal*. Descent is commonly unilineal, and so is succession, though they do not always follow the same rule. Inheritance is mainly unilineal, though it often has some bilineal aspects.

In modern England the principles are mainly patrilineal — a person takes his father's surname; titles go to sons or failing them to brothers, and there is a strong tendency for the inheritance of property, particularly of land, to go in the male line. Unthinkingly we often regard this as the 'natural' method. But there is no intrinsic reason why continuity of groups and of privilege should not be effected through the female line. In fact, it is done in a great variety of non-industrial peoples, especially in Melanesia, in North America, in central Africa, and in parts of India and Southeast Asia. Sometimes the matrilineal principle is accompanied by a system of *matrilocal (uxorilocal) residence*, that is, the husband goes to live with his wife and her relatives. The workings of the matrilineal principle may be seen in examples from central Africa and from Melanesia.

Among the Bemba of Zambia descent is matrilineal. A man takes his mother's clan, and speaks of his village of origin as the place where his mother and matrilineal uncles were born. He traces back his ancestry mainly on his mother's side. With a man of chiefly rank it is typical to find the ancestors remembered for thirteen generations on the mother's side, and only for two on the father's. Succession is also matrilineal. The office of chief passes first to the dead man's brothers, next to his sister's sons, and then to the children of his sister's daughters. A chieftainess is succeeded by her sisters, maternal nieces, and granddaughters. There are few forms of wealth to be inherited, but in former times a man received a hereditary bow on the death of his maternal uncle. But nowadays money is often divided between a man's own children rather than between his nephews. In former times a man lived in the village of his wife, and occupied an inferior position there in the early years of married life. After two or three children had been born he could move with his wife to his own village. Children over three are still sent to their mother's mother to be brought up, and in olden days were largely in the power of the mother's father or brother, who had rights to their services. He could even offer them as slaves in compensation to some family which he or his kinsfolk had injured.

The picture here presented is something very different from the type of organisation to which we are accustomed. But just as in our society the formal patrilineal rules still leave room for important social relations with a mother's family, so also in a matrilineal system the father and his kin are not ignored. When the anthropologist speaks of a matrilineal or a patrilineal group or system, he speaks only of dominant principles. Audrey Richards, on whose account of the Bemba we have drawn, makes it very clear that the father and his matrilineal group have an important part to play. A man is called by his father's name and not by that of his mother's brother. Again, in native belief there is an intimate magical connection between a man and his wife and child, so that a father has an important rôle to perform in the ritual life of a young child. In these early years, isolated in a strange village, he is still called the owner of the child and considered essential to its well-being. Sentiment of children for father is often keen, and though their mother has been long divorced, grown men and women will make a long journey to visit their father and give him presents. Even in former times a father had definite rights over his children. He had to be consulted about his daughter's marriage;

103

he had the right to distribute the payment received for her, and the son-in-law worked for him and not for his wife's kinsfolk.

At the present day contact with European culture has greatly increased the power of the father. The demands of wife and children for clothing and other European things are growing rapidly, and a father who, through wage-earning, makes his children gifts of this kind can maintain his rights over them more easily than of old. The exodus of men to work in the copper mines has diminished the practice of serving for one's bride, and also of matrilocal residence. Hence the power of the wife's relatives has been lessened. Again, the ignorance of Europeans of how the matrilineal system really works, and to some extent their prejudice against it, has tended to act in the same way. Audrey Richards stated 'young men believe it to be more English, and therefore more fashionable, to claim their father's clan instead of their mother's, and some missions have definitely encouraged this change.'

Any system which attempts to emphasise too exclusively one side of the family as against the other carries within it the seeds of discord. We have seen among the Bemba a duality of rights and privileges and a balance which, though formerly weighted on the matrilineal side, is now tending to go down on the patrilineal side. In the Trobriands the two principles seem to have been more directly in conflict, even apart from any stimulus afforded by European contact. A good example is

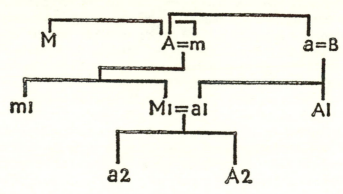

Fig. 3
(Capitals indicate males, small letters females.)

104

given by succession to chieftainship and its implications as described by Malinowski. The Trobriands system is such that when a woman marries, her brothers have to make heavy annual contributions to her husband's food supply. On the other hand, though marriage is patri-local, a brother is the guardian of his sister and her children, the latter being his heirs. In the diagram (Fig. 3) A is a chief. His rightful heir is his sister's son A1. To him he must hand on the rule of the clan, his canoes, yam houses, and other valued property, and also his know-ledge of magic. But we have referred earlier to a father's interest in his child. A chief or other man of rank will give to a favourite son all that he can safely alienate from his heirs – plots in village lands, privileges in hunting and fishing, precedence in dancing, and even some of the hereditary magic. But such gifts and privileges excite the resentment of the sister's sons and must cease at the father's death. Cases where such resentment has expressed themselves in bad rela-tions between son and sister's son are not at all uncommon. But by making use of a recognised type of marriage the chief can assist his son to retain these benefits. This is a cross-cousin marriage, that is, a union of the children of brother and sister. The chief A marries his son M1 to his sister's daughter a1. The result is that M1 now has to be supported by A1 with annual gifts of food. Moreover, the taboo which prevents a man from knowing anything about the sex relations of his sister stops A1 objecting to the marriage. (Traditionally, this may be arranged by infant betrothal, and he is not even old enough to understand what it means.) Not only does M1 secure the economic assistance of A1, but he is also entitled to friendly treatment. Among other things he can live in his father's village, that is, the village from which he would normally go when A1 enters into his inheritance. Moreover, though A1 succeeds A in time he himself will be succeeded by his own sister's son A2, that is, by the son of M1. The net effect is that a kind of intermittent patrilineal succession goes on within the framework of the matrilineal system. The cross-cousin marriage thus gives an opportunity for a resolution of the conflict between the two principles. (It has been questioned whether in fact such Trobrian mar-riages were ever frequent, but the example illustrates an ideal type of many such actual kinship arrangements elsewhere.)

Types of kinship group larger than the individual family have been mentioned incidentally in the examples discussed earlier. Such

105

larger kinship groups usually play an important part in non-industrial society. Their members frequently co-operate in agriculture; land is often owned by these groups and not by individual families; marriages may be arranged between them, and they make a common appeal to their ancestors. There are many kinds of such groups. They vary in size, in the principles of descent which govern their membership, in the ways they use to demarcate the group and give it individuality, and in the type of marriage rule which their members must observe. Anthropologists are not yet fully agreed as to how all these types should be classified, but one scheme which represents a collective opinion of a number of British anthropologists is given in *Notes and Queries on Anthropology* (Royal Anthropological Institute, 1951).

In discussing kinship groups, one must draw a distinction between those which meet sporadically for personal occasions and those which exist as continuous entities. A funeral assembly is an example of the former when people from the father's group, the mother's group, the father's mother's group, and the mother's mother's group, may all attend – on the bilateral principle. They are oriented in relation to a particular person – the *ego* of the anthropologist's conventional kinship charts – and since this person is now dead they may never meet again as a group in any other capacity.

The other type of group persists generation after generation, keeping its essential individuality as a separate unit in the society, losing some members, but gaining others. It is normally unilateral and unilineal, consistently relying for membership on ties of people with their fathers or their mothers, but not both. Basic advantages in these unilineal groups seem to lie in their economic and social functions. The holding of land, and the transmission of titles, privileges, and material goods, tend to be facilitated when either the male or the female line is followed alone. Two important varieties of such groups are *clan* and *lineage*.

A clan is a unilineal descent group of major order in a society, acting as a unit in a system of similar groups.[5] The separate clans in a system are usually named, and are often distinguished symbolically by associations of a totemic kind with natural species. Clans usually have some corporate functions of a political or ritual order, and may play a very important part in community life. Clan members nor-

106

mally regard one another as kinsfolk, though they may not be able to trace their relationship genealogically. Frequently, they express their relationship in rules of exogamy – whereby a member must marry outside his clan. Formerly exogamy was taken arbitrarily by anthropologists as a critical feature of demarcation in identifying a clan system, and distinguishing it from other sets of major kin units. The existence of a rule of exogamy affects the constitution of the group by strengthening the unilineal principle, as well as by enforcing complex relationships of an economic and ritual kind. It also ensures that fresh people join the domestic circle. But in many respects non-exogamous descent groups, whether unilineal or not, have much the same functions as have exogamous groups in other societies. They too are therefore called clans. Clans are found in many parts of Africa, Australia, Melanesia, and North America. They have been identified also in China, but not with precision. Clanless societies include the occidental states (save for a few survivals of reduced function, such as Scottish clans) and most oriental civilised states, as well as the simplest primitive societies, such as the Andamanese, the Senoi and Semang of Malaysia, the Eskimo, some Indians of California, and the people of Tierra del Fuego. Many more communities, such as most Polynesians and some central African tribes, also have no clans. (The Tikopia have a system of non-exogamous clans.)

A *lineage*, meaning primarily a line of descent, is now taken also to mean a unilineal descent group, all members of which trace their genealogical relationship back to a founding ancestor. If the lineage system is patrilineal (or agnatic), the members consist of men, their children, and their sisters, and trace their descent through males, normally to an original male ancestor. If the system is matrilineal, the members consist of women, their children, and their brothers, tracing descent through females, normally to an original ancestress. Such groups are usually exogamous. Groups of lineage type usually tend to form sub-groups by division, in what has been called segmentation, fission, ramification, or branching. In regard to this branching process, these groups have been termed *ramages*, a name which links with the metaphor that some of these systems use, that they grow like the branches of a tree. (It seems more convenient now to reserve the term ramage for a kin-group of a lineal type, but ambilateral or

107

cognatic, i.e. the members trace descent from a common ancestor, but do not follow an exclusively male or female line, and moreover do not practise exogamy.) Attempts have been made to distinguish lineage groups according to their size, position in the segmentary system, and functions. But there is as yet no uniform classification, and it seems better to recognise simply major and minor lineages in general, separating varieties of these by reference to their empirical aspects where necessary.

To some extent kinship and local organisation coincide. The elementary family is nearly always the most important constituent of a household. Members of an extended or expanded family frequently share a group of dwellings or live closely together, as in the joint family still common in Malabar and some other parts of India. But the members of the larger scale kinship units often do not live together *en masse*, and rules against incest inhibit any complete exclusiveness. A village may contain members of several clans; and a clan may have its members scattered through many villages. We tend to find then that whereas the smaller kinship groups function chiefly in the domestic field and in co-operation for everyday economics, the larger kinship groups tend to be concerned mostly with ceremonial occasions, such as marriage, initiation, and death, or with religious ritual.

Where there are no corporate unilineal kin groups of size, as in parts of central Africa or of the Solomon Islands and New Guinea, the principle of local affiliation is of prime importance. The village or group of hamlets is here the major social unit, made up of people who have attached themselves freely to a headman, to whom many but by no means all are related genealogically. Where, as in parts of Southeast Asia and Polynesia, there are corporate kin groups but not unilineal, residence is commonly the factor determining to which kin group a person shall belong.

A striking feature of kinship is the way in which terms which we regard as appropriate only to near relatives are used very widely, even perhaps through the whole range of a clan. A man may call by a term equivalent to 'brother' not only his father's sons, but his father's brother's sons, and other first cousins, and indeed all the men of his own grade of kinship as far as he can trace relationship. This is what is called the classificatory system of kinship terms. It must be pointed out at once that though the term may refer to a whole set

108

of people, this does not imply that the people are regarded as all standing in the same relationship to the speaker. Thus, a man who calls his father's son and a distant fellow-clansman both 'brother' knows very well the difference in their relationship to him and can explain it. Often the native language has terms such as 'true' or 'real' or 'own' to distinguish close from distant kinsfolk. Moreover, a person treats his own brother in many ways quite differently from his clan brother. He will borrow things more readily from his own brother, perhaps joke with him more freely, discuss certain family secrets with him, help him more readily, and mourn for him more keenly.

The classificatory system presents some curious usages. In some societies it is the custom for a man to call his father's sister's son – his first cousin – 'father', and for this man to call him 'son' in return. At one time there was a theory that this was due to an ancient type of marriage of the father's sister's son with the wife or widow of his mother's brother, which would make him the legal father of the mother's brother's children. Nowadays, however, it is seen that this and similar customs are due to social or economic reasons. For instance, Fortune has shown that in Dobu a man calls his father's sister's son 'cousin' until his own father dies. After that he calls him 'father'. This is not because the father's sister's son marries the widow, but because he inherits the village land, the name, and status, and even the skull of the dead man, who is his mother's brother. One does not need, then, to suppose some extraordinary form of marriage to explain a dramatic change of kinship terms.

It is not possible to discuss in detail other important principles of social structure. But a reference may be made to two of these principles. Occupational specialism is important in some societies. Even in the most undeveloped from a technological point of view, where there is little room for economic specialisation, a magician or medicine man often stands apart. In parts of Africa blacksmiths form a special group, and the practice of their craft is surrounded with a great deal of ritual. This reflects itself in their social position; sometimes they are honoured and treated with respect, sometimes they are regarded as pariahs and subject to social disabilities.

Another important social principle is that of status. Status has been defined in many ways. But it is convenient to regard the social status of a person as his position in a social system, represented by the rights and privileges he enjoys and the obligations or duties he should perform. Status can be *achieved*, by individual effort, or *ascribed* (accorded) by society to individuals because of their inherited place in a particular kin group or their other prior claims to recognition. Achieved and acquired status are contrasted by the elected chairman of a tribal committee compared with the hereditary chief of the tribe, or a shaman who becomes distinguished by his special charismatic powers contrasted with an hereditary clan-priest. But these two kinds of status often shade into one another. Statuses are frequently graded on a scale of prestige. The term rank is used for such grading in the political and ritual fields – though it is given a more general meaning too. When a graded system of statuses is of general operation in a society, affecting many spheres of social activity, it is termed a system of social stratification. Here, each stratum or layer in the grading scheme is composed of people who fill much the same position in the social structure. Important general types of social stratification are *estate*, *class*, and *caste*. In a system of estates, exemplified by a feudal type of society, the various social strata are distinguished particularly by their legal position relative to one another, and also by differences in their social functions and privileges and their ways of behaving. In a class system the primary distinguishing feature is often taken to be economic position and function, though phenomena of class are often identified also over a much wider field. In a caste system, though difference in economic function, particularly occupation, is regarded as extremely important, the distinctive character is the way in which the differences between the strata are expressed and defined in procedures with a high symbolic, even ritual content – as for instance in the idea of pollution.

To the differing magnitudes of the legal, economic, and ritual elements in these systems are related differences in the degree of social mobility. The ability to move from one stratum to another in the system is an important feature of a stratified social structure. Even the most rigid system, such as caste, is not entirely closed or unalterable, whatever be the overt rules and beliefs. In the Indian system, for example, new castes or sub-castes are added from time to time by including hitherto pagan groups now converted to Hinduism, by socially integrating a group such as Parsis or Jews whose basic religious tenets are different, or by the fission of an existing group, the members of which have previously inter-dined and inter-married. Again, caste groups at times have managed to elevate themselves within the system as a whole by making social use of economic advance, demanding and receiving improved status as their wealth and power have increased relative to those of other groups in their social field. And in modern times emigration and diversified employment have allowed some men to obliterate their former status and assume a new one, by claiming membership of a caste group to which they did not formerly belong.

An important aspect of social structure linked with status is the political dimension, expressed in the structure of authority and control of resources, including manpower. There is great variety in political structures, from simple assemblies of elders or councils of many tribal communities to chiefs and rulers of Polynesian islands, African emirates or Malaysian sultanates, and representative institutions of modern democracies. In the more developed societies elaborate mechanisms exist for the maintenance of power and control of the productive capacity of the community. These mechanisms are expressed and protected by practical and symbolic means, often of a highly ceremonial order. For instance, traditionally a Muslim African Emir in northern Nigeria after prayer at the end of the fasting period (Ramadan) came on horseback before his palace, and the heads of his districts and administrative departments, with their followers, galloped up before him on their horses in a spectacular charge. This dramatic demonstration was in token of fealty to him, and was accompanied by dancing and presentation of gifts. As I have myself seen (Plate 15) the Emir's horse was richly caparisoned and he wore a black velvet cloak with silver embroidered head-dress, distinguishing him from all others present. The chiefs doing homage to him, and attendants, wore multi-coloured robes, with a riot of red and yellow, and fans, trumpets and drums enhanced his position. The social structure in its political dimension is thus given visible form.

NOTES

1 The concept of social structure has involved much debate. Most anthropologists use it, as I have done here, to refer in a fairly straightforward empirical way to the main principles which can be identified as responsible

for the behaviour of people in a given society. Some of these principles may be expressed as overt rules, which may be even ideal norms rather than actual patterns of behaviour; and some anthropologists would restrict the idea of social structure to these ideal rules. Some of these principles may be of a more abstract order, possibly unrecognised by members of the society. Some anthropologists, especially from a Marxist standpoint, stress such features of 'inner structure', such as the character of basic power relations arising from control of economic resources but veiled by notions of free contract. Related to the idea of social structure but with much wider implications is the structuralism of Lévi-Strauss which reveals how notions of categorical opposites – such as 'raw' and 'cooked', 'up' and 'down' – can serve a people as conceptual tools for the formation of abstract ideas and of propositions relating to them. 'Structure' in this sense is highly abstract and is concerned with the laws inherent in the logic of attributes perceived by the human mind in basic thought. (See Cl. Lévi-Strauss, *Structural Anthropology*, London, Merlin, 1963; *The Savage Mind*, London, Weidenfeld & Nicolson, 1966; Cf. E. R. Leach, *Political Systems of Highland Burma*, London, Bell, 1954.)

Some anthropologists, as I have done, make a distinction between social structure and social organisation. While social structure refers to the principles or norms guiding people in a society, social organisation refers to the arrangements involved in their acts of choice and decision as individuals adapting to the behaviour of one another and the external circumstances.

2 Since about 1952, when Tikopia young men began to go abroad to work, they have tended to cut their hair short. As Tikopia young women too have come more into contact with the world outside they have tended to grow their hair longer. Dancing and funeral customs have been affected correspondingly. Contrariwise, young men in western society have tended to wear their hair long.

3 There are sectors of society, e.g. in the West Indies in which the rôle of a father in the family is often minimal, the responsibility of children being borne by the mother, who is unmarried. But in other cases, even though no legal tie exists between the parents, they maintain a regular household, in a state which has sometimes formerly been described as 'faithful concubinage'. Moreover, in such conditions the ideal in status terms for the woman is commonly that of marriage.

4 The idea that a man fertilises a woman, who thus conceives a child, is not unknown to the Trobrianders; they have heard it from missionaries and anthropologists as well as from their neighbours, the Dobuans. But traditionally, they have denied it strongly.

5 British writers use the term *clan* for patrilineal as well as matrilineal groups of this type. American writers formerly used *clan* for matrilineal groups only, and *gens* for patrilineal groups, though R. H. Lowie and others have used *sib* for both. G. P. Murdock has proposed clan as a term for kin groups based both on a rule of descent and a rule of residence.

112

CHAPTER FIVE

The Regulation of Conduct

IN our discussion of economic life and social organisation we have seen that physical and biological facts, nutritional urges, blood relationships, age similarity, and common residence give a basis for social ties, and link people together in groups. But such factors can also produce disharmony and conflict: clashes between old and young; quarrels between neighbours; sexual jealousy; bickering over inheritance; opposition of economic wants. Every human society seems to be at once unified by the centripetal force of the common interests of its members and riven by the centrifugal force of their individual and sectional interests.

Our problem in this chapter is to consider what regulates the conduct of people in their group life, how individual behaviour is guided along certain channels, apathy overcome, and conflicting interests kept in check. The rules of conduct in any society are difficult to classify, but, broadly speaking, they comprise rules of technique, of taste and fashion, of manners, of morals, of law, and of religion.

A distinction can be drawn in theory, and to some extent in practice, between what people actually do – the 'rule' in the sense of a statistical average – and what they ought to do – the 'rule' in a normative sense, of a standard to be aimed at. In practice these two kinds of rule tend to coincide. What most people in fact do is felt to be what every one should do. It can be said to be the rule in England for the majority of people to eat three meals a day, to wear foot-covering in towns, to sit on chairs, and to marry only one spouse; we look upon this as the natural way to behave, needing no regulations to make us do so. Yet if we think about it, we see that behind each of these customary ways of behaving is an 'ought' of one kind or another. Children are not allowed by their parents to skip a meal without comment; a wife is expected to get breakfast and dinner for her husband and he to have lunch out; restaurants look askance at people who want meals at 'odd' times. To go barefooted in a city is eccentric; to sit on the floor may offend one's hostess; to marry more than one wife brings down condemnation by Church and State. Yet in some other societies, as we have seen in earlier chapters, people eat but one meal a day, go with naked feet, sit on the floor, and marry several wives, and are expected by others to do all these things. Men, unlike other animals, have a wide choice between different ways of behaving in a given situation, and make their choice largely for social reasons. They are guided in what they do by the opinion of their fellows, and ideas of what it is proper to do – by values.

In some spheres, however, there may be a wide gap between the rule which ought to be followed and what is actually done. In spite of the fact that the English pride themselves on being a tolerably law-abiding people, returning travellers often fail to declare to the customs authorities goods that they have obtained abroad; motorists often exceed the speed limit; and business men evade income tax. The Christian theme of love for one's neighbour is in strong contrast to commercial dealing, restrictive tariffs, and the building up of armaments. The discrepancy between the legal or moral rule and the actual practice is not merely due to ignorance, negligence, or individual self-interest. Loyalty to others, ideals of efficiency and practicability, beliefs in the unfairness of the law, conformity to public opinion, all help to provide a set of additional standards which allow individuals and groups to justify their departure from the admitted ideal.

For those interested in the life of Man in society a number of questions arise. Are there in other societies similar rules for the regulation of conduct? If so, how far are they clearly formulated by the people? How far are they kept, and if they are broken, for what reason? What is the reaction of other people to such a breach? Is there any machinery for enforcement of the rules? And if they are, on the whole, effective, whence comes their power? And finally, why do such rules exist at all? Let us attempt to answer at least some of these questions.

It has sometimes been vaguely said that simple hunting peoples, such as African pygmies, are like children, obeying no rules and following their own fancy. Or, again, that they have their own customs which they follow blindly, and that when once they have decided to do something they can be moved by no argument. And, further, that many of their customs are 'queer', that is, one can see no sensible

114

reason for them, and therefore one is reduced to classifying them under the heading of taboos. We shall see how far these popular opinions are true. In the first place, it can be said quite definitely that in all known human communities social order is preserved to some degree. There is no wholesale violence or unrestrained aggression. But, on the other hand, there is no passive conformity to an ideal of the good of the community. The social order is not an unconscious process; it is an affair of rules, and of keeping or breaking them according to a variety of individual interests, and responding to conscious obligations and training. In each society these rules form a system. In most African or Oceanian societies, for instance, they are not codified – there are no Ten Commandments, or any set scheme of numbered injunctions, nor are rules always expressed as abstract principles. It is often difficult to draw out a general formulation, and one may hear a rule uttered only in reference to some actual incident. By such means a great deal of the education of young people is done.

Though we have spoken of many non-industrial societies as being simple in their organisation and in their technical achievements, this does not mean to say that their rules of conduct are few and simple. The model *Handbook of Tswana Law and Custom*, compiled by Schapera, for instance, covers the rights and duties of citizens of the tribe, marriage law, rules for the relations between husband and wife, parents and children, and kinsfolk; the law of property relating to land tenure, cattle, and other domestic animals, household and personal effects, and inheritance; the rules for barter, sale, loan, and gift of goods, and the performance of services; and for a variety of legal wrongs against the person. Careful studies of other societies – by Gutmann on the law of the Chagga of Tanganyika, by Malinowski on Trobriand law, by Hogbin on the law of the Polynesians of Ontong Java, by Thurnwald, Adam, Gluckman, Arthur Phillips, and others on indigenous law in Africa and the South Seas, and by van Vollenhoven, Korn, Ter Haar, and others on the Adat law of Indonesia – show an equally complex fabric of rules of behaviour. Thus we see that it is superficial just to say that behaviour is regulated by 'custom'. 'Custom' is a much overworked word and comprises a number of different types of rule which vary in application, in strength, and in the kind of response which any breach of them brings forth. We can see in alien societies rules of the same order as those which we

115

distinguish as manners, ethics, morals, law, and religion, granting that our own distinctions are not always very consciously and clearly made.

The popular notion that technically underdeveloped peoples lack all the gentler forms of social intercourse is very wide of the mark. Codes of manners seem to exist in all societies, and a half-naked 'savage' may be just as polite as a civilised European. For instance, a Polynesian once brought me a gift of green coconuts on a hot day. When I drank, and pressed him to drink also, he refused, though he admitted he was thirsty. He explained courteously, 'In this land one does not partake of a gift that one has brought, lest people say, "One who eats his own present".' Here, then, is a delicacy of attitude that is at least as refined as our own.

Sometimes local manners seem even excessive. Roscoe mentions that the Baganda in olden days had a code of etiquette which included fulsome greetings and thanks even to those met by the wayside. When Europeans were seen they were politely thanked for being well dressed, or two of them might be thanked for walking in step – even though the 'thanks' might be only an empty phrase!

Even where the greeting does not conform to our usages none the less it follows rules of etiquette. The Tikopia or the Malay peasants do not say, 'How do you do?' on meeting a person on the path, but ask, 'Where are you going?' This is not inquisitive or rude, but is the convention. It may be answered either by a factual reply or by the vague words, 'I am going for a stroll.' If anything, it is as sensible as the English 'How do you do?' which is not now intended as a genuine inquiry about the state of one's health, even though a naïve stranger may reply in those terms. The important thing in these modes of greeting is not the overt meaning of the words, but the fact that words are uttered, that some verbal bridge is thrown across the social gap between people coming into fresh contact.

For the European entering an alien community, conformity to local manners is one of the best ways to begin co-operation. Asians or Africans often think that Europeans are rude because they make no attempt to adapt themselves. A shaping of one's own manners to those of another community is one of the easiest sacrifices to make; it does not mean giving up the more fundamental values involved in a moral code or religious belief.

Alien peoples have their own ethical and moral judgments too. Persons are regarded as good or bad, actions as right or wrong – though not infrequently a single vernacular term does duty for a range of ideas for which we have separate words such as 'correct', 'good', 'right', 'proper', and 'virtuous'. The fact that alien codes of morality differ must not, however, cause us to say that some are on a 'higher' level than others. The truer view is that each is adapted to particular social conditions, and should be judged according to its efficiency in maintaining social order.

By the 'immorality' of alien peoples is usually meant nothing more than that their codes are not ours. This is clearly seen in the case of sex relations. In western Europe chastity before marriage is at least a moral ideal to those who follow the orthodox conventions. In some Oceanic communities such as the Manus of the Admiralty Islands, or the chiefly families of Samoa and Tonga, this is also the case. But in a great number pre-marital sex intercourse is not only common but also regarded as right. To call this immoral ignores the fact that, like other social activities, it has rules to regulate its occurrence and its consequences. It frequently exists side by side with standards of opinion which prescribe the type and degree of intercourse to be indulged in, which are critical of frequent changes of lovers, and which place strong penalties upon conception, or at least upon the birth of a child outside wedlock. Our moral judgments in this sphere often tend to overlook social realities. Condemnation of pre-marital intercourse overlooks the fact that, as Malinowski has shown for the Trobrianders, it is often an essential element in the process of education in sex matters before marriage, and of experiment in the choice of a mate. It meets to some extent the difficulty caused by a wide gap between puberty and marriage.

The much-criticised institution of child marriage in India has been defended by Hindus on the ground that one function of it is to prevent the dangers of pre-marital sex relations of girls. It has been stated to me by missionaries that one difficulty which has arisen from the success of their efforts in stopping child marriage, with its admitted evils of too early bearing of offspring and exploitation of the young, has been that now cases occur of girls bearing illegitimate children, with all the consequences of shame and family friction.

Our own conception of morality is complicated by the fact that it

117

is so closely bound up with religion. Relations before and outside marriage are contrary to Christian rule; marriage itself is a sacrament as well as a legal contract, and in England we have recently seen how closely the law of divorce is scrutinised by the Church and interpreted in accordance with religious dogma. The frequent association which the Christian Church makes between sex and sin is, as we have seen, not found in many non-western societies. So also, in general, morality is quite often separate from religion. It is rare to find among the sanctions of right conduct in a tribal society the belief that good and bad people go after death to separate destinations or conditions, which are regulated according to the moral quality of their behaviour on earth. Much more frequently rank, wealth, and social condition in this world give different passports to the next.

When we turn to the sphere of law in non-literate societies, we are confronted by difficulties of definition. There is usually no specific code of legislation, issued by a central authority, and no formal judicial body of the nature of a court. Nevertheless there are rules which are expected to be obeyed and which, in fact, are normally kept, and there are means for ensuring some degree of obedience. The classification of these rules and the definition of law in African or Oceanic societies have become at times a matter of some argument.

The simplest basis of classification is that of the practising jurist who tends to equate law with what is decided by the courts. On this criterion most African or Oceanic peoples have no *law*, but simply a body of customs. This classification is of practical importance when such societies are subject to the government of European powers, and where it is a problem as to how far the traditional rules controlling behaviour should be taken into consideration. This point will be dealt with later in Chapter Seven. But for the anthropologist studying alien societies this formal juridical approach is not very helpful, because it considers custom only in relation to what use the courts can make of it, and does not examine how it operates where there are no courts. This is not, however, the only juridical pont of view. The sociological jurist, examining the concept of law from a broader standpoint, is interested in all kinds of rules that exist in a society and in the problem of their functioning. This is more in line with the anthropological approach. The major difference of opinion between anthropologists is between those represented by Malinowski, who would include in

118

the study of law all types of binding obligation and any customary action to prevent breaches in the pattern of social conformity; and those represented by Radcliffe-Brown, who would restrict the sphere of law to the entry of the force of a politically organised society. An intermediate position has been taken up by Godfrey Wilson in his study of Nyakyusa law and custom. He took as the criterion of legal action the entry into an issue of one or more members of a social group who are not themselves personally concerned. In this tribe it is common, for instance, for disputants to take their quarrel to a senior kinsman, a friend, or a respected neighbour for adjudication, and this Wilson treated as part of the tribal law. This would be treated by some anthropologists as private arbitration of a non-legal kind, and, indeed, to take only this element of procedure as the criterion of definition of law seems somewhat arbitrary. A great many societies in Melanesia and Australia, where there is no such appeal to a person outside the dispute, would on this basis have no law. If a definition of law which would separate it from 'custom' is thought necessary, then it would seem to lie in bringing together a number of elements – rules; the degree to which they are obligatory; the degree of obedience to them; the degree of precise formulation of them; the character of the sanction for them; the type of authority with which they are enforced; and the acceptability of this authority. Law is a function of all these together, and not of any single one of them. It relates particularly to the sphere where the rules are closely formulated, highly obligatory, the sanction for them is strong and frequently negative, and the authority by which they are enforced is of an organised kind. This in effect is the standpoint of the jurist. But the need for such a definition does not seem to be great for sociological purposes. Whatever be his basis of classification the sociologist still has to remember that for the understanding of law in this sense he must be prepared to examine all these elements in the wider sense, and to specify the degree to which each enters into the situation. If a system of European law is intelligible only by reference to the changing practices of the people, their system of ethics, their institutional structure, their judges' ideas of what is 'reasonable', and non-legal factors which lead them to keep it or to break it, how much more must this be so in the case of a non-western people without such a clear-cut formal scheme?

Consideration of this array of means of securing control of the behaviour of people raises the questions of the source of these means, of how judgments are passed, and by whom they are carried out. A highly organised legal system recognises a division into legislative, judicial, and executive functions – represented in England, broadly speaking, by Parliament, the courts, and the administrative services, including the police. Such a clear-cut division is not a common feature of a system of law in a tribal society. The main body of rules does not originate through the act of any specific body appointed for the purpose, but is believed to have existed from immemorial antiquity. The force upon which their power rests is that of the tradition of the society which is the nearest equivalent to the 'sovereign' in the Austinian sense. Sometimes, however, by a general agreement, new rules are introduced, or an old rule interpreted to meet changing conditions, or again, common practice in such conditions imperceptibly comes to be regarded as the rule which should be observed. Schapera in his study of Tswana law gives a very clear exposition of the sources of their rules of conduct. The Tswana speak of the main body of their laws as having always existed, from the time that Man himself came into being, or as having been instituted by God or by the ancestor spirits. A further source of law is given by the judicial decisions of the tribal courts which in their judgments recognise and strengthen the obligatory character of most existing rules, but occasionally by distinguishing between cases give rise to new precedents. A third and mainly modern source of their law is given by the decrees of their chiefs who have the power to abolish outgrown usages or issue new regulations for the better conduct of tribal affairs. In many tribal communities, however, there are no chiefs, and even where they exist they have no specific legislative functions. Nor again is there often any organised judicial body which can give an impetus to changes in the system of rules.

Judicial machinery, then, frequently does not exist as a separate department of tribal law. The passing of judgments is done not as an organised affair, but through the unorganised exchange of opinions among the people discussing the event. In aboriginal Australia, when an important rule is broken, there is no formal calling together of an assembly to discuss the matter, but it is canvassed by the group of adult men, who are normally in close contact with each other. To de-

120

cribe their common discussions as a legal council would be an over-statement; they certainly discuss the merits of the case, they make concessions for extenuating circumstances, and they may arrive at a decision, but there is no formal procedure, and the decision emerges out of the general talk and is not a formal pronouncement. Moreover, it is not necessarily the elders who play the most influential part. Younger, more vigorous men, assertive in personality, may dominate the opinions of the gathering, and may often precipitate a decision. Much the same is true of complex politically organised societies such as Tikopia in Polynesia. Here the decision of a chief has a final authority which may not be gainsaid, and often guides conduct or causes punishment to be visited upon an offender. But this decision, though it is controlled to a considerable extent by the advice of other men of influence and by public opinion, is not taken as the result of any formal judicial council. It may spring from his own immediate perception of an event, or from informal discussion, or be almost forced upon him by some party that goes to him and pleads for him to issue a command. The non-literate societies in which the formal judicial apparatus is most highly developed are mainly in parts of Africa. Here a council of elders, or a chief in council, or a court, may proceed in quite a formal manner, admit plaintiff and defendant, call witnesses, pronounce an explicit decision, and order the execution of the judgment.

Along the same lines a body of executive officials to carry out legal functions is often lacking. In some communities there are persons who act as 'police'. In Tikopia, for instance, the brothers and close cousins of a chief bear a special title – and are recognised as being primarily responsible for carrying out his decisions and for keeping order in the land. They can even serve as protection and aid to individuals who have fallen under the wrath of another man of rank. Hence their title of *maru*, 'shelterers', because they afford shelter to the people as a tree casts its shade as a relief from the sun. In many societies, however, a judgment is put into affect by some of the people immediately delegated or even self-appointed from the social group as a whole.

In this chapter we are concerned primarily with the general nature and functioning of the means of regulating conduct, the forces of social control rather than the content of the rules in themselves. A

121

number of important problems, then, including an analysis of family law and the law of property, of civil and criminal injuries, and of the procedure of adjudication and the theory of motive and responsibility, cannot be explained here.

Let us now consider the working of rules. It is a commonplace that although rules usually have some penalty attached to their non-observance, they are not observed merely because of the penalty. In non-western as in western society, men do not abstain from stealing simply because of the punishment for theft. Consideration of this question brings in the question of sanctions. There is no clearly agreed definition of what is meant by a sanction. The older juridical idea derived from Austin was that a sanction was the penalty probably incurred in case the rule was disobeyed. The modern jurist has broadened this to include the reward for keeping the rule, and considers sanctions as the conditions calculated to render the law effective. If these conditions are interpreted widely this is essentially the anthropologist's view. He feels it necessary to take into account not only those conditions immediately connected with the law itself, such as fines, rewards, possibility of prosecution, respect for Parliament, etc., but also the general conditions of the community life – and these not on the simple plane of acquiescence of the governed, recognition of benefits to be gained, or the inertia of habit, but the active forces of public opinion, education, the moral view of obligations. The action of any individual in respect of a rule is governed not only by his immediate personal interests and the degree of temptation which he has at the moment felt, but by his recognition of what a variety of people in contact with him will say, think, feel, and believe, and by what he knows them to have done in the past. The conditions which make the law effective may then be restated as those activities and responses of individuals, whether expressed in the name of the society or not, which tend to govern the behaviour of a person in respect of a rule, and to maintain order and equilibrium in the social system.

One can view these sanctions in a number of ways, which represent cross-classification. Some are *personal* to the individual, as the complicated pull of his own interests, his inertia of habit, and the fullness of his recognition of the nature of the issues; others are *social*, such as domestic or public approval or disapproval, retaliation, punish-

122

ment, etc. Another classification could be into *immediate* and *ultimate* sanctions; the former arise directly from the nature of the rule, such as the punishment following on its breach; the latter are of a more general character, such as the fear of being talked about, or the loss of future benefits. A further classification adopted by Radcliffe-Brown is of a more precise and factual kind. After distinguishing organised from unorganised sanctions, this proceeds from ethical and moral sanctions through sanctions of retaliation, restitution, and punishment to those of a ritual order. Those of restitution and punishment alone are considered as legal sanctions.

Without pursuing any of those classifications further, we may list here a number of the most important sanctions, particularly in non-industrialised societies. Some of them, of course, function also in industrialised societies.

The sanction of public opinion is always extremely important. Usually unorganised, it sometimes assumes an organised character, as when in western society presentations are made for saving life, or meritorious exploration, or social service. Sometimes public opinion can be expressed in a crystallised form through the agency of proverbs, which have greater weight than a purely individual opinion at the moment. Among the Maori proverbs played quite an important part as a stimulus to action or a check upon it. Ridicule in some societies may assume a set public form as in the taunting songs of the Eskimo or of the Tikopia. Theft in Tikopia is dealt with by tongue-lashing, and sometimes by physical violence if the culprit is known. If he is not, then the bereft owner may compose a dance song embodying his views of the thief with slighting allusions, and get it chanted in full chorus at the public dances on the beach. Primarily this relieves his feelings, but to some extent it acts as a sanction by shaming the thief before any who may know of him.

Another type of sanction often of great importance is that of reciprocity. He who breaks a rule or does not do his duty may find himself on short commons at a later date, or without necessary labour, or blocked from achieving some valued object which would give him prestige. By breach of the rule for immediate gain he wastes his assets for the future. Realisation of this plays a large part in keeping many a man on the straight and narrow way of social conformity. That whole system of values which may be comprised under the head

123

of tradition, inculcated by the complex processes of training and learning, is also of vital import. The law is often kept not because it is the law, but because it is thought right to keep that kind of rule. As we have seen, non-literate people have their ethical formulations, and rely upon them.

Another group of sanctions is of the kind popularly known as superstition. This is usually a slipshod term to describe someone else's religion. But more precisely it may mean a faith in the supernatural which we regard as irrational. A taboo in the concrete sense, a bundle of leaves tied to a pole, with a backing of supernatural force, is a common means of protecting property in society in Oceania. Sometimes this taboo is believed to punish an offender through its own magical power, sometimes through action by spirit beings or ancestors to whom it has been dedicated. Fear of supernatural punishment is a sanction even though no material token is set up. In many communities incest is held to be punished by the intervention of the ancestors of the guilty pair, who visit them or their offspring with sickness and death. In Tikopia this sanction and that of public opinion act alone with no sanction of any physical kind. Persons who commit incest are not punished by their social group as they are, for instance, in many African communities. A third sanction of the supernatural type is that of sorcery. Malinowski has shown that in the Trobriands the power of a chief, which is an important factor in the preservation of law and order, is maintained quite considerably by his employment, or the fear of his employment, of sorcerers. Among the Australian aborigines the fulfilment of obligations of ceremonial exchange is facilitated by a number of factors – recognition of future economic and other benefits to be obtained, wish to conform to the traditional pattern, or a desire to maintain one's reputation as a 'good trading partner'; in addition failure may involve the need to fight, and it is believed that a bad partner may have sorcery levelled against him. Ritual practices to avert the wasting sickness and death believed to be consequent on such sorcery are not infrequent. A further type of sanction is that of retaliation by physical violence upon an offender. Among the Tswana retaliation is still sometimes allowed in cases of assault, particularly on a woman. The court will instruct the injured woman to inflict upon her assailant an injury of the same kind as she herself received. Then again there is the sanction of restitution, where the breach of a rule means that the offender must hand over property to the offended party. Such a type of sanction is extremely common in African tribal law. Finally, there is the penal sanction where the organised force of the community working through the machinery of a chief, a court, or a council punishes an offender.

All these sanctions do not work with equal effect in every society. In some the weight of public opinion is highly mobilised to secure conformity to rules, and organised restitution or punishment do not play an important part. Supernatural sanctions, again, enter much more throughly into the regulation of conduct in some societies than in others. There is not space here to examine the different types of conditions which give these sanctions their differential weight.

It must be observed that just as the types of rule to be kept vary from one society to another, so also does the classification of behaviour as offences. In Europe, for a man to go through a marriage ceremony with a woman while he is still married to another is an offence in law and a sin in religion. But, as we have seen in Chapter Four, it is not only permissible, but is a socially desirable practice in most Muslim countries and in many other societies. The African belief in the rightness of polygamy has created difficulties for the Christian Church in Africa, and has even been partially responsible for the secession of local Christians from the parent mission. In England, to enter private property without leave is a trespass against which the owner can take action in law. But in Tikopia, to plant crops on the land of another person without having obtained leave is regarded as quite permissible, and the owner is not expected to have a grievance provided that a basket of the crop is given to him at the harvest. Where the same type of act is classified as an offence, the immediate sanction against it may vary considerably. The intentional killing of another person is in western countries a criminal offence, visited with punishment, sometimes by death. But in many parts of Africa the traditional rule has been that homicide within the tribe is a matter not for punishment of the killer, but for the paying of compensation by him and his kin-group to the relatives of the slain person. Here, again, the difference in the sanction applied has been a cause of difficulty in the application of western law to such communities. In other communities, again, the immediate sanction does not take the form necessarily of punishment of the guilty person, but of retaliation upon his kinsfolk if he himself is not available. This concept, crystallising in the form of the blood feud, has also increased the complexity of governing an African people by western standards. Sometimes, again, the immediate sanction for damage to a person or his property is not the exaction of compensation, but the *lex talionis* of classical times – the 'eye for an eye and tooth for a tooth' of Mosaic law.

It is clear that at the initial stage of introduction of western law to a non-western community, as with the establishment of colonial rule, there may be a conflict of sanctions. One result of this is often to produce an increase of certain types of offences, which by local rule were punished much more severely than by European law. An example of this is adultery. In Malaita in the Solomon Islands the commission of adultery was normally visited with death by spearing. Under European government, an aggrieved husband can only sue for divorce or demand compensation for alienation of affection. This to the Malaita people seems insufficient, and it is said that adultery has grown more common thereby. Another result of alien rule is that acts have now become offences which were formerly not so, and people become lawbreakers in the eyes of the European governments, though they may be right according to their own traditional rules. Examples of this are the avenger of a kinsman's murder who now becomes a criminal instead of the executor of justice; and a defaulting labourer who, in fulfilling his obligations to attend some tribal ceremony, breaks his contract with his European employer. Consideration of such cases leads us to see that the conflict between tribal ethics and compulsions on the one hand, and European law on the other, may be a very real one, disturbing to the life of a people who have respect for their traditional rules. In the past this has been a strong argument for a close examination of the forces of social control in colonial communities, and for an attempt to incorporate into the system of administrative justice as much as possible of the local concepts.

In a traditional society unaffected by western contacts there is no conflict to any great extent between the different types of sanction at work; the whole scheme is fairly well integrated and consistent. In western society, however, with its great complexity of many different types of social groups with different immediate backgrounds, such conflict is only too apparent. What is felt to be right, or at all events permissible, to an individual may clash with what the law prescribes or forbids. An outstanding example of this was the widespread breach of the Volstead Act in the United States of America, when prohibition was in force. Large sections of the population manufactured, imported, and consumed alcoholic liquor contrary to the law. This wholesale disregard of the law obviously did not mean that a large percentage of Americans suddenly displayed criminal tendencies, but that operating against the legal sanction were strong sanctions of what may be called a moral kind. In another sphere, historically there has been the conflict of sanctions in regard to divorce, and the remarriage of divorced persons, in Britain. What the State permits the Church is reluctant to allow, and the position is complicated still further by the fact that to many people the religious sanctions are not of much weight. Many are of the opinion that to lay cardinal emphasis upon technical adultery as the grounds for divorce, and to disregard such factors as temperamental incompatibility, is to overlook one of the most important elements to successful marriage. Moreover, it produced this anomaly, that persons who might have no wish to seek sexual satisfaction outside marriage were forced to commit or to appear to commit at least one act of adultery in order that the marriage might be dissolved. Ethics, law, and religion at variance created a situation of disharmony which has had no exact parallel in traditional African or Oceanic societies.

There is one difficult problem to which the anthropologist has yet been able to give no satisfactory answer. In all the bewildering complexity of rules which we have seen existing in a range of societies of varying technical development and economic and political differentiation, is there any common basis to be found? Is there anything that can be termed 'natural' law? The answers that have been given by philosophers and by the exponents of religious doctrine have often been quite definite. But these answers depend on certain initial assumptions concerning which there is by no means general agreement. Moreover, certain of these assumptions are definitely declared to be outside the province of science. One such assumption is that the value of human life is intrinsic, that every individual has a *right* to live, and that only in cases of extreme offence can the State

127

decide to abrogate this right. On this assumption practices of infanticide, which are not uncommonly resorted to as an escape from difficult social situations such as threatened embarrassment with an illegitimate child, or pressure of population on food supplies, are condemned. This judgment may be passed even when no other remedy for the difficulty can be immediately seen. In consequence people who practise infanticide are arraigned as criminals and reprobated by the Church, even though in local eyes they have committed no wrong. Yet in western society the logical implications of this assumption are not rigidly followed through – except in the case of a few groups such as the Quakers. In what is deemed to be a situation of national necessity the taking of human life becomes not an offence, but a praiseworthy action. The State does its best to compel it by conscription, and the Church blesses the arms and stigmatises the foe. Here, then, we see in our own circumstances a supreme need to abrogate the moral law, which we deny to others.

To turn from war to sport. The arguments about the merits and demerits of fox-hunting in England are too common to restate here. But there is one appendage to it which is of interest. In former years there have been several cases in which the Royal Society for the Prevention of Cruelty to Animals has prosecuted officials of hunts 'for causing suffering to a fox by allowing it to be unnecessarily worried by hounds'. In some of these cases the official of the RSPCA appears to have said that he did not object to fox-hunting as such. The general assumption here is that pain should not be inflicted upon animals where it is avoidable. Here we see the curious feature of singling out for legal action one single aspect and moment of what must on any honest examination be recognised as a painful process for the fox in its entirety. It has been claimed that the fox enjoys being hunted, except presumably when he is actually being torn to pieces, but as yet we have no evidence of this. The presumption is, in fact, all the other way. The conflict of sanctions between the established institutions of fox-hunting and all its values, what the law allows and prohibits, and the humanitarian views of many sections of the people gives rise to a position which it is hardly possible to defend on grounds of its consistency. In one defence of such a case it was stated that to say of any MFH that he caused suffering to a fox would be very distressing, and that in this instance the Master's kindness to

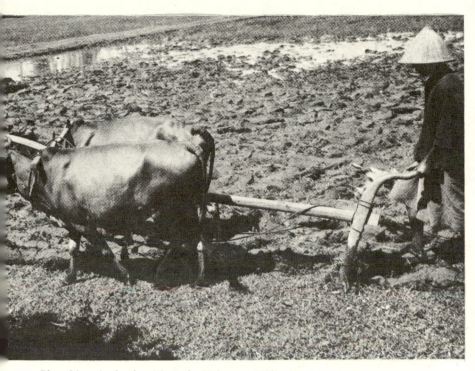

11 Ploughing rice lands with cattle, Kelantan, Malaysia

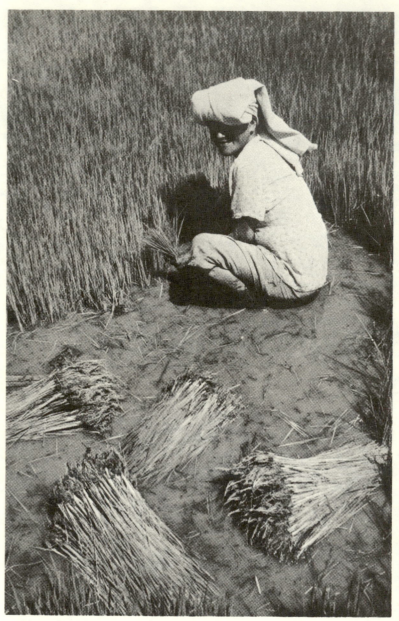

12 Transplanting rice seedlings, Pahang, Malaysia

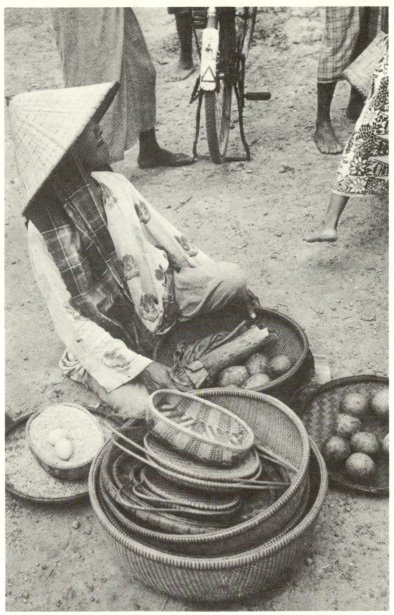

13 Selling fruit and vegetables in the market, Rabaul, New Guinea

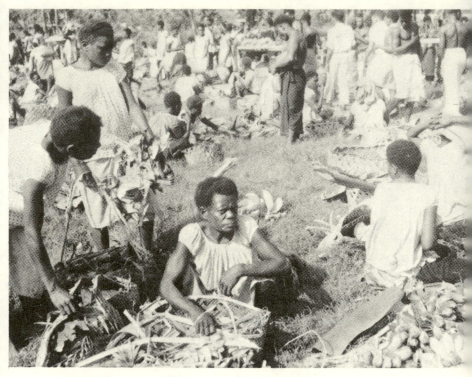

14 Selling baskets and fruit, Trengganu, Malaysia

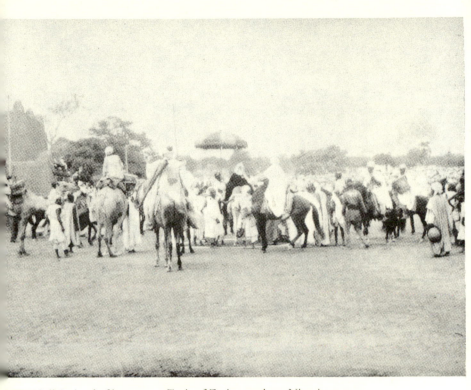

15 Sallah ritual of homage to Emir of Zaria, northern Nigeria, 1945

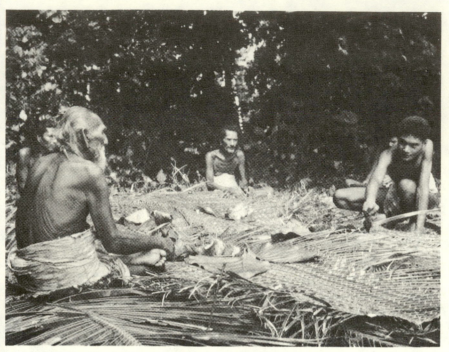

16 Cooking in an earth oven for a funeral feast, Tikopia

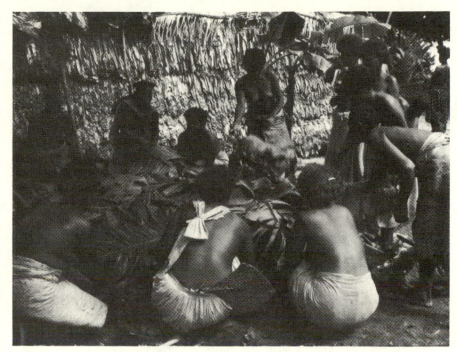

17 Pouring a libation to gods and ancestors, Tikopia, 1952

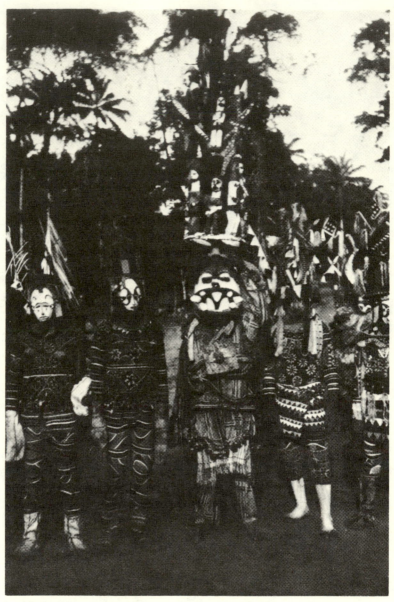

18 Masked dancers impersonating female spirits and spirits of large land and water animals, Onitsha, eastern Nigeria, 1945

animals was 'simply notorious'. Instead of this intellectual refusal to see the inconsistency involved, it would be more logical to say that a fox-hunter in his pleasure in the sport, which might be justified on other grounds, is willing to forgo up to a point his humanitarian interest in the avoidance of pain.

The scientist searching for some common denominator in social rules, for some basic universal quality which might be termed an absolute, is faced by much inconsistency of this kind, by much failure to examine the bases of assumption and to employ these assumptions in a logical way in actual life. Where, perhaps, the anthropologist of the future may be able to see some basic quality in the variety of rules for the regulation of conduct, is by engaging in a more precise search for the conditions of social efficiency. If men are to live together in groups, there must be some conditions for their co-operation and mutual contact. Physical violence must be restrained, aggression kept within bounds, and machinery provided to decide between interests which conflict or appear to conflict. As yet the results of this search have been expressed only in very formal abstract principles largely of an *a priori* kind, and need much more inductive, empirical inquiry to establish their validity.

CHAPTER SIX

Reason and Unreason in Human Belief

In earlier chapters we have dealt with the sphere of secular activities as against sacred activities, or temporal as against spiritual power. We have been examining what Durkheim has called the Profane aspect of life. In nutrition, technology, economics, law, and the activities of family and kinship we have seen man in diverse forms of society as a reasonable being. His solutions to the vital problems which confront him, though they are often different from ours, appear to us as alternative rather than illogical. In a non-western society one can recognise the formulation of principles and judgments about the external world which seem to us to be rational, that is, founded upon premises which appear to conform to what we know to be true of the physical universe, and which follow logical processes of thought in their application to concrete situations.

Lévy-Bruhl, it is true, has held that primitive thinking is pre-logical, i.e. is based upon a different kind of link between the observer and the object from that in the case of civilised peoples. This link he called 'mystic participation'; the 'savage' does not view the external world in what we would regard as a dispassionate way, but sees it through a kind of emotional haze in which trees and animals partake of something very like a human quality. His thesis has not received general agreement. It is admitted to have been a great stimulus to the investigation of thinking in different social circumstances, and in a way is true of certain aspects of the attitude to nature in totemism and kindred institutions. But Lévy-Bruhl has overlooked or whittled down the mass of evidence in which non-western peoples, on their own statements and by their actions, take a line of procedure of which we would approve. As I have shown, if a Polynesian is making a canoe, he selects a light wood for the outrigger float, he streamlines the hull, and may even flatten that side of the hull which is nearer the outrigger in order to counteract its drag, just as a European boat-

130

builder would if he built such canoes. This is a striking illustration of their rationality in technical affairs. It is true that such peoples often do not use the precise categories of classification that we do. In conformity with the fairly limited range of their experience, and the absence of a class of intellectuals who live by probing into meanings, they do have fewer categories. But they use others which serve their own purposes effectively, and which represent rational principles of classification.

It has been necessary to stress this point in order that in our discussion of magic and religion it should not be imagined that thought in a non-western context moves primarily on an emotional level, and that action is substantially governed by irrational factors. The person who is supposedly being instructed may even apply critical analysis of a rational order to views presented to him, and which he regards as not well founded. In the *Missionary Notices* of 1829 it is recorded that some missionaries talked to some Maori about the resurrection of the dead, when the following remarks were made by the Maori: 'How many persons have already been raised from the dead? Did you see them?' Being answered in the negative they laughed heartily, saying, 'Oh! Indeed! You only *heard* of it from someone else.' When ideas of this order are not backed up by their own traditions and current tales, people are often ready to adopt this disconcerting commonsense attitude.

In all the major aspects of traditional Polynesian activity beliefs in the supernatural have played a large part. If we follow our Polynesian canoe builder carefully we will find that side by side with his technical operations he performs other acts not dictated by purely technical principles. He believes that his canoe-working tool is controlled ultimately by a spirit being; he believes that through this being it has the power of killing borer in the timber; he dedicates the vessel to gods and ancestors whom he invokes to give it speed and seaworthiness, to send wind, or calm the rising waves, or bring fish. When we call this supernatural belief, we do not mean that the things believed in are necessarily regarded by the believers as being 'above' Nature, but that they do not form part of what our experience has led us to classify as *natural* forces. In action they are supplementary to ordinary human effort. It has been already mentioned that such beliefs in the supernatural – as taboos, or the power of ancestral spirits – can act as forces of social control. It is important to recognise that though the basis of a belief may be an illusion, the belief itself may have real and valuable effects. We might thus classify such types of belief and action as 'irrational', or in modern idiom, 'non-rational', not because they are illogical in their inference from certain premises, but because the premises themselves are not valid by our scientific analysis.

To base these beliefs on feelings of awe, mystery, or on a 'religious thrill' is too simple an explanation. Their close integration with practical affairs, with economic wants, and with the critical periods of human life, cannot be accidental, and it seems, therefore, as if they have emerged in response to some fundamental human needs. But to say that they are primarily due to what the magician or priest makes out of them is too simple. An 'exploitation' theory of magic or religion ignores the reality of the beliefs held by the practitioner himself, his own deep conformity to traditional values, and the pressure often put upon him by his community to carry out his spiritual ministrations.

Science and magic ordinarily represent the two poles of reason and unreason, but it is not easy to draw a rigid line between the rational and the irrational spheres of human activity. If, for instance, we take the question of the relation of technical knowledge to magic, we find a number of graded types of attitude and of activity in which elements of both are present. Some types of curative 'magic' employ substances which do seem to produce a real effect. Others indulge in rational experiment. On the other hand, the practice of science itself is not entirely free from an irrational prejudice for certain theoretical views, from the refusal to give due weight to evidence which runs counter to a favourite assumption, and from the almost mystic reverence with which many people view a statement that is supposed to have the authority of 'science' behind it.

But let us consider magic as commonly accepted, that is, a rite and verbal formula projecting man's desires into the external world on a theory of human control, to some practical end, but as far as we can see based on false premises. A broad classification of magic in terms of these practical ends, whether the promotion of human welfare, the protection of existing interests, or the destruction of individual well-being through malice or the desire for vengeance, is given in the following table:

Aim and Sphere	Social Aspect
A *Productive:* Magic of hunting. Magic of fertility, planting, and harvest in agriculture. Magic of rain-making. Magic of securing a catch in fishing. Canoe and sailing magic. Magic for trading profit. Magic of love.	Performed either by private individuals for themselves, or by specialist magicians for others or the community as a whole. Socially approved. A stimulus to effort and a factor in organisation of economic activity.
B *Protective:* Taboos to guard property. Magic to assist collection of debts. Magic to avert misfortune. Magic for the cure of sickness. Magic for safety in travelling. Counter-magic to C.	Performed as above, and socially approved. A stimulus to effort and a force of social control. *Sorcery:* performed as above, sometimes socially approved, sometimes disapproved. Often a force of social control.
C *Destructive:* Magic to bring storms. Magic to destroy property. Magic to produce sickness. Magic to bring death.	*Witchcraft:* sometimes attempted, often doubtful if actually performed; and sometimes of imaginary occurrence. Classed as morally bad. Provides a theory of failure, misfortune, and death.

This classification does not necessarily follow vernacular linguistic distinctions between types of magic, which are often of a more concrete kind, with separate terms for the individual types mentioned. Sometimes, again, the productive magic may be described simply by the general word for 'formula', while special words are used for protective and destructive magic.

Analysis of a magical act reveals several characteristic features. There is a definite practical aim to be achieved, and there is a human performer of the magic. This person, by the conditions of the magic itself, has frequently to be in an appropriate condition – he may have had to be abstinent from sexual intercourse, he may have refrained from eating certain foods, he may have to be in solitude, or to be clothed in a certain way. In the practice of the magic itself there are normally three elements: the things used; the things done; the things spoken. The first element is represented by the *instruments* or *medicines*; the second is the *rite*; the third is the *spell*. Let us look at each of these in turn. The instruments used are often primarily of a technical kind. A canoe-builder who wishes to kill borer in the timber cuts gently with his adze on the wood and recites a form of words to destroy the insect. But sometimes the instrument is not of technical significance in craftsmanship. Such is the quartz crystal of the Australian curer of sickness, or the pointing-bone of the central Australian death-dealing wizard. In Africa great use is made of 'medicines', magical objects or compounds often fashioned or concocted from trees and plants. A list of medicines known among the Zande would probably number several thousands, though any individual knows and uses only a small fraction of these. The leaves of bulbs are eaten raw, or boiled in water with sesame and salt and eaten. Parasitic plants have whistles and charms manufactured from them. And from creepers are made medicines to enclose gardens and for winding around a man's wrist for protection. In many Bantu languages the word for 'medicine' is the same as or akin to the word for 'tree'. It is alleged that some of these medicines have properties which do produce the desired physiological effect, but most of them appear to be inert. Medicines used in witchcraft, or believed to be so used, often contain exotic substances such as the brain of a crocodile, the flesh or the fat or the afterbirth of human beings. Usually special conditions have to be observed in the gathering of these medicines – just as for the materials of the witches' cauldron in Macbeth. Often these medicines are kept in special containers which themselves may have some magical virtue, or at least be an index to the kind of medicine they contain. Among the Bemba medicines are frequently contained in the horns of antelopes, in small gourds, or little cloth bags. In the gourds and bags magic of good luck, of popularity, or protection against illness are usually carried, and in the small *duiker* horns is carried hunting magic, but in the horns of bush-buck evil magic is usually placed. This animal has a bad reputation among the Bemba. It is believed to be an evil spirit, and is taboo as food to chiefs and pregnant women. With medicine in such a horn a wizard would be able to lay the spirit of his victim and send it back to the grave.

According to African theory the power of magic is believed to reside in the medicine. In this it differs from most Oceanic magic, where the power is believed to lie in the spell.

The rite has almost an infinite variety, but in essence its function is to bring the magic and its object into contact. Sometimes the rite and the technical procedure are one, as when a Tikopia fisherman recites his formula to the fish as he lowers the line. He uses no medicines nor any act of a distinctively ritual kind. Sometimes, however, a specific act is performed with no practical value, as when a Trobriand canoe-builder sweeps the gunwale with a bundle of light grass as he recites the spell to give the canoe lightness and speed.

The verbal element in magic is extremely important – so much so that Malinowski regarded it as the fundamental constituent and the believed source of magical power. There are said to be a few magic rites when no spell is recited, but it is possible that the magician does here at least express his formula in thought. In many communities such as the Maori, the Trobrianders, or the Dobuan, the form of words is thought to be fixed and invariable, so much so that a mistake in the recital may spoil the effects of the magic. In others, however, particularly in Africa, the form of words is variable, and consists rather in a conversational address to the medicine to perform its work, the magician modifying his phrases at his discretion. Where the form of words is fixed – the spell proper – then certain conventions usually obtain. The words are often alliterative and onomatopoeic, suggestive by their sound of the end desired. Again they convey analogies to what is wanted. When the red turmeric pigment is being manufactured in Tikopia some of the phrases used refer to the blood-red hue of the flowers of the coral tree and the ginger, to the bright red of fish, and to the red-fringed leaves of a plant. Figures of speech, and references to mythology are common, and again some of the words are cryptic in form and archaic, so that they have no meaning apart from their particular magical context. As Malinowski insisted, they are not meant to convey information, but to be a mode of action and an expression of human will. The formula is, then, a translation of the urge of human desire into words, and the rite and spell are the spur of the hand and voice to the forces of Nature.

One obvious question which must strike anyone who sees or reads of magical practices must be: Why do they exist when they rest upon principles which often run counter to those we know to be true? Why has the performer not perceived the fallacy of his magic? Long ago Edward Tylor pointed out four reasons for this. First, some of the results aimed at by magic do actually occur, though for other reasons, or because there may be some real virtue in what is done or in the

135

medicines used; secondly, in some cases trickery may be practised by the magician to deceive his fellows – though on the whole the magician believes as firmly in his magic as do others; thirdly, positive cases count for more than negative cases – even in our own experience we often ignore things which run counter to theories in which we believe; fourthly, there is the belief in the existence of counter-magic. If a rite fails to produce its end, then it is argued that the proper conditions have not been observed, or that someone else has magically conspired against it. A good example of the way in which the theory of magic puts up new bulwarks against an attack upon it out of its own very principles is seen in the case of the attempted resuscitation of a dog by some Papuan sorcerers in 1931. This was a test staged at the request of a government officer. To the Europeans who saw it, the test failed; the sorcerers were shown to be pretentious liars. But the sorcerers themselves still believed in their powers; they argued, first, that the conditions in which the experiment was performed were not propitious; secondly, that the dog had been killed in a manner which gave them no opportunity of working on the remnant of vital essence, which it was essential for it to retain in order to be brought back to life. The impression of other Papuans present was that the experiment would have succeeded, and that the dog was actually coming back to life when over-zealous interference by a village constable spoilt the result, and again reduced the dog to a lifeless condition. From this it can be seen that the belief in magic and the practice of it cannot be simply put down to stupidity or credulity, but must be explained in terms of the acceptance of certain assumptions about the nature of things and logical argument from them. The strength of magic lies in the strength of the beliefs that these assumptions are valid. Why should they be so firmly held? To understand this it is necessary to see what is the rôle of magic in the social life.

Magical practices are not performed simply for their own sake; they have in each case a direct practical aim, and they are associated with other human activities of what we should call a rational kind. If we were to analyse in detail the relationships of productive magic to the enterprises with which it goes hand in hand, we should see that it normally performs certain functions in these enterprises. These have been admirably analysed by Malinowski. In the first place, productive magic may throw over the technical operations to which it is attached a cloak of sanctity, increasing the seriousness with which they are performed, and even threatening punishment if they are neglected. Again, productive magic often sets the pace for the actual work. According to the rules of the magical scheme, various stages of the work must be performed at due intervals to allow the magic itself to be carried out in proper sequence. Magic, then, can have a useful organising power. A more general function which has been stressed by Malinowski is that magic tends to make for confidence in those who employ it. The sphere with which it purports to cope is essentially that of the unknown and the unpredictable – of rain and drought and insect pests in agriculture, of wind and storm and perils of the sea in sailing, of the desires and feelings of a trading partner, or the vagaries of the heart of one whom one loves. Productive magic asserts man's power over Nature, and allows him to go forward with his aims in the conviction that through his own efforts he can command success. From this point of view magic cannot be overthrown by any mere demonstration of its fallacy. It is too deeply intertwined with the fundamental springs of human emotion.

This psychological theory of magic just mentioned must be taken as true only in a general sense in any given case. It may be impossible to demonstrate, and there are situations in which magic is not used though human knowledge cannot predict the issue. The Tikopia use no love magic; the Manus of the Admiralty Islands use no sailing magic, but rely upon their own skill and courage to face a rising storm; the Trobrianders, on the other hand, use both these kinds of magic to a high degree. Magic is, then, only one form of cultural response to situations of uncertainty. Other responses may be a reliance upon a beneficent God, a reliance upon the theory of probability – which is another name for science, or a simple fatalism which rejects both science and God. The reason for the different distribution of the magical and other responses in different types of society is something which as yet anthropology and psychology has not been able fully to explain. An answer commonly given, that it is due to historical processes, still leaves unsolved the problem of why the pattern of action took just this historical form.

Protective magic also has its obvious functions. Granted the belief in its efficacy, it serves to defend the rights of individuals, and though it may not produce any real effect upon offenders, it does serve to give sufferers a means of assuaging their feelings of outrage and their desire for vengeance. As Evans-Pritchard has pointed out, for the Zande a belief that sorcery is an instrument of punishment, and can produce death in offenders, is a comparatively harmless method of enabling people 'to let off steam'. It causes less disruption in the society than the use of the spear.

We may now turn to an analysis of destructive magic. Let us first compare the pattern of destructive magic in several societies. Destructive magic among the Maori consisted essentially in destroying some part of the victim's clothing or hair or nails or even his excreta with the recital of a powerful spell. Among the Zande of central Africa *mangu* or witchcraft is a kind of emanation from an imaginary material substance in the bodies of some persons. It is thought to be capable of being diagnosed by oracles in the living, and is said to be discovered by autopsy on the dead. To the Zande ordinary magic and witchcraft are of quite a different order. In comparing the magic of these two societies we see that among the Maori there is no use of medicine, that destructive magic and productive magic are of the same generic kind, and that destructive magic is actually practised and relies for its success on the use of objects associated with the victim. But whereas the productive magic of the Zande is very similar to that of the Maori, Zande destructive magic has an additional category to the Maori type. Side by side with the sorcery which is actually performed and follows a special technique, is witchcraft, which does not require either formulae or exuviae of the victim, and is not actually capable of human performance. This duality in the sphere of destructive magic is commonly found in Africa as well as in Australia and parts of Melanesia. It does not, however, appear to exist in Polynesia.

Among the Daly River people of Australia, according to Stanner, two varieties of destructive magic have been actually practised: the rite to bring on storms and damage one's enemies; and the burning or burying of personal exuviae to cause sickness and death. Also, there is a belief in and a great terror of *mamakpik*, the stealing of a living man's kidney fat with his resultant rapid decline and death. This presents the features of the Zande *mangu* in that it is never witnessed, and though a person may be accused of practising it he never admits to doing so, and its activity is diagnosed essentially by its supposed

138

effects. But unlike the possessor of *mangu*, the practitioner of *mamakpik* had no supposed organic peculiarity of his body. In rare cases an attempt has actually been made to steal kidney fat in the prescribed fashion, but has naturally failed. In some parts of Melanesia there is a strong belief in a type of destructive magic, some of the cardinal features of which are physically impossible to carry out; yet there are people who actually profess to perform it. Such is the *vele* of Guadalcanal and the *vada* of south-eastern New Guinea, in which a magician is believed to daze his victim, extract vital organs, miraculously close the wound, and resuscitate him for a short time, though he cannot name his assailant and dies soon afterwards. The major difference of this from the Australian *mamakpik* is the existence of men who purport to practise this magic.

There is in all this destructive magic a set of common elements, though the emphasis upon each may vary from one community to another, and a fairly clear distinction can be drawn between one type, the practice of which is imaginary, and another type, where some ritual is actually performed. It is common to describe the first type as witchcraft and the second as sorcery, though these terms are not always uniformly so used.

A great deal of what we have said about magic also applies to religion. It is founded on assumptions from beyond the sphere of reason, it uses manual rites and verbal formulae, and the condition of the performer is frequently held to be proper to the success of its appeal. But a number of points for distinction between them have been put forward. As examples we may mention Frazer's formal criteria, which have been widely adopted, of magic being an assertion of man's control over Nature by the commanding power of the *spell*, and religion as his reliance on spirit powers through the appeal of the *prayer*. Then there is Malinowski's functional criteria of magic being a simple belief in the definite effects of man's power of using spell and rite, limited in technique and directed to a definite practical end; and religion as a complex set of beliefs and practices, united not in the form of its acts or subject matter, but in the function which it fulfils, self-contained, and finding its fulfilment in its very execution. Piddington, again, takes a cross-classification of religion as the ideology of the supernatural, and magic as its application to practical affairs, so that in activities which are ordinarily regarded as essentially reli-

139

gious there would be on his definition a magical component. Other writers have stressed the difficulty of drawing such a distinction, and prefer to speak of the magico-religious sphere as a whole. Linked with this are two further points. The practices of magic are frequently individual, with one person opposing his interests and his emotions to those of his fellows, creating disharmony rather than resolving it. Those of religion are essentially social, often partaking of the ritual of a church, with the basic aim of adjusting individuals to their social environment, leading them to find peace within themselves, and reconciliation with others. From this comes the moral classification of magic as something frequently bad from the social point of view, and religion as something good and socially valuable. We speak of black magic but never of black religion.

Using any criterion singly the distinction between magic and religion can be easily drawn. But when they are considered in conjunction the two spheres cannot be so clearly demarcated. The table opposite shows that elements ordinarily considered to be magical can be found in rites ordinarily considered as religious, and vice versa.

Within the Christian Church prayer may be used to secure immediately practical benefits. Not so many years ago a rural dean blessed the nets of a whitebait fleet of the Thames estuary before the fishing began; the Mayor of the town helped to pull in the nets, supplies of the catch were sent to cabinet ministers and three hundred guests attended the whitebait supper organised by the Chamber of Trade. In 1935 an Austrian cardinal blessed all motor-cars assembled at St Christosen in lower Austria, the ceremony being attended by the Austrian Minister of Trade and the local Government. This strongly resembles the consecration of the implements of production, with the ensuing ritual feasts, that take place in many a simpler society, and is frequently classed as magic. These prayers often represent the claims of sectional as well as individual interests. When prayers for rain are recited in our churches, for instance, the answering showers are not an unmitigated blessing to all members of our society. On a wider scale sectional interests are still further represented by the national alignment of different sections of the Church in time of war. In such ways religion can be just as practical, just as closely linked with technology and economics and with the interest of specific groups, as magic.

I Elements in situations commonly regarded as		PRIMARILY MAGICAL ELEMENTS WHICH ARE COMMON ALSO IN RELIGION.
	Affirmation of human control of supernatural.	
	Spell commanding obedience.	Compulsive power of words.
MAGICAL	Rites using magical substances (medicines) which have their own powers.	Virtue of material and other symbols (the Cross), images, idols.
	Belief in supernatural power (*e.g. mana*).	Utilisation for sectional or individual ends.
	Manipulation for individual interests.	
II Elements in situations commonly regarded as		PRIMARILY RELIGIOUS ELEMENTS WHICH ARE COMMON ALSO IN MAGIC.
	Reliance on extra-human aid.	Control through spirit agencies.
	Prayer appealing for aid.	Material interests of group.
RELIGIOUS	Rites using symbols, offerings, and sacrifices.	Prayers for rain.
	Belief in spiritual beings.	Blessing of technical equipment and of economic methods and adjuncts.
	Group participation, as e.g. in a church.	

The basic attitude in prayer is that of appeal. But many of the forms of prayer by their phraseology alone are commands, and it has even been held that persistent prayer will inevitably bring a response. The idea that God answers prayer is in a way an assertion of the power of the spoken word to bring the results we desire.

In many Oceanic societies what is ordinarily classed as magic can contain elements ordinarily regarded as religious. In Tikopia, for instance, when a man is fishing with a rod and line on the reef, he recites a formula commanding the fish to come to bite on the hook.

He addresses the fish alone and brings in no spirit being. But he does not merely order the fish to obey, and he does not believe that the mere virtue of the words in themselves constrain obedience. He talks to the fish as he would to a human being, he cajoles them with tempting offers. He believes that they hear and appreciate his words, though he is not sure of this, since fish live in the depths of the sea, and he cannot observe them. But he also calls upon spiritual beings, his ancestors and guardian deities, to assist in bringing the fish to him.[1] Here command and entreaty, belief in his own power of 'spellbinding', and in the power of his spirit helpers are so closely intertwined with his practical situation, that to separate out the magical and religious elements involved would be to tear the formula apart, phrase by phrase, and almost word by word. Moreover, these same spiritual beings are invoked during the great fertility ceremonies, which represent the high point of the Tikopia ritual life, or during crises of life such as initiation, sickness, and death, and which could only be called relgious on any ordinary classification.

If we look back now at our table we see that we have to deal, not with magic and religion as two exclusive spheres, but with a variety of different combinations of the elements we have discussed. In so far as a distinction can be drawn on broad lines it is in describing certain acts, and the situations in which they take place, as primarily magical at one end of the scale, and primarily religious at the other. In between lies a sphere in which the elements are so closely combined that the institutions may be termed magico-religious or religio-magical. In practice such intermediate types are commonly found.

The argument about this classification has been complicated by the view, formerly held by many anthropologists and still held by some, that the belief in spiritual beings is more complex than that in supernatural power and human control; that it is higher in the evolutionary scale of human progress and later in development. From this point of view difficulties are solved by speaking of any combination of elements as a transition stage. In view of our ignorance of the historical development of religious institutions over much of the world, this should be regarded as an evasion of the problem rather than a solution of it.

We may now turn to an examination of the character and function of those aspects of belief and practice which can be termed primarily religious. It is not today necessary to prove, as Tylor had to prove half a century ago, that all known peoples, however primitive, have a religion. This 'religion' may not be of the type to which we are accustomed, but it is none the less real and fills an important place in their lives. It may include acts that shock and horrify us – head-hunting, cannibalism, human sacrifice, mutilation of the body. It may include beliefs that seem childish and absurd, in the powers of stones and trees to move and to talk, in veneration for animals and birds, taboos against simple ordinary habits, beliefs in contaminations which the human body can suffer. Yet it includes, too, beliefs of con-siderable imaginative power and even of beauty, cults of fertility and of vegetation, personification of natural phenomena, and tales about them. Strangely assorted as they may seem, these things can be found linked together in the religious life of a single people. Fresh from a western, especially Christian training in the idea that the real essence of religion is in a unique inner feeling, in a personal experience, of a high emotional kind, it may be difficult for us at first to give sympathy and understanding to religion of another kind. In some of these reli-gions, such as are found in North America, a unique personal exper-ience in the form of a vision, often of a high emotional quality, does occur, but it is lacking among many non-western peoples. Belief is firmly held, but it is taken for granted and not made an object of catechism, and an individual proves his allegiance by his acts and his participation in cults, not by his inner convictions. The practitioner of such a religion would agree with those Christian apostles who argued that faith must be demonstrated by works. Again, segregation of the individual and private communion with the unseen powers is not usually a feature of a tribal or analogous religion. The most com-mon rite is one of public assembly. So much is this true that Durkheim has given its extreme expression in his theory that religion essentially connotes a church, and that the idea of God is really that of society deified.

It appears that in every society men believe in the existence of spirit entities and spirit powers which influence human activity. This impressed Tylor so much that he based his minimum definition of reli-gion on what he called animism, and described as a belief in spiritual beings. When we think of a religion we usually think of a god or gods. But a non-western religion frequently concentrates upon beliefs in spirit powers which it is difficult to classify in this way. In Australia religious belief is concerned with ideas of pre-existing spirits, which, often through the action of superhuman tribal heroes, become embodied in living animal and plant species and in natural objects. These are sometimes linked with human artifacts such as the bullroarer, which are treated as sacred, and become the focus of rich ceremonial and artistic practices concerned with fertility and the crises of life. In addition, as on the Daly River, there may be a belief in ghosts, and in spirits of the hobgoblin type, which come as apparitions and startle people. In most areas of Australia one supernatural being, the Rainbow Serpent, takes the dominant place as a culture-hero to whom are attributed many of the most important creative feats. From the eastern tribes there are reports of a supernatural being of the order of a god, known as Baiame or Darumulum, but the rôle of this being in the religious life is not altogether clear, and such a concept seems to be lacking in other areas of Australia that have been well studied.

A broad survey of spirit beings recognised among most peoples reveals two principal categories: those regarded as human in origin, and those which are non-human, though they may have human attributes.

The beliefs in the spiritual beings, powers, or principles derived from Man are diverse, and discussion of them is difficult, since the categories of them found in various parts of the world do not coincide with our own nor are they the same in all societies in any given area. We distinguish broadly the body and the soul. But we have other concepts which represent different facets of the human individual. We speak of a person's *vitality*, thinking of something partly physiological and partly psychological. We speak also of his *personality*, as a psychological expression, though it often amounts to the equivalent of his social aura, the kind of impact which the projection of his individuality makes upon others. Something of these ideas runs through the ideas of many peoples. But since our idiom of speech and thought expresses itself in distinctions such as those of natural from supernatural, and psychological from spiritual, we are apt either to superimpose our own categories directly upon those of alien peoples, or to regard these alien categories as confused, perhaps even to the people themselves. We attempt to render their terms as 'soul', 'per-

144

sonality', 'sub-conscious', or to classify their beliefs as a theory of multiple souls.

What in effect they have done is to take different facets of human experience and of the immaterial side of man's activities, and to combine them in ways somewhat different from ours. In translating the terms which classify alien belief into our own language we have usually to be content, then, with merely rough approximations. It is not that we are incapable of understanding their beliefs, but that the luggage in our portmanteau of terms is differently distributed from that in theirs.

It is impossible to list here all the facets of human experience and individuality which, say, African or Oceanic peoples distinguish. But we may refer to four of the most general. These are an immaterial essence or vital principle, a dream counterpart, a shadow counterpart, and that element which survives after death and may be termed the soul, or the ghost.[2] Often, however, some of these coincide.

The immaterial essence of human beings is a kind of invisible counterpart of the body, vague and formless, like some unseen fluid. On its well-being that of the body is believed to depend. If it is abstracted from the body then sickness follows, and if it is not restored the body dies. It is often thought to be subject to sorcery. For this reason the ancient Maori in leaving a seat frequently made a scooping motion with his hand behind him in order to gather up any portions of his immaterial essence which a sorcerer might work upon to his undoing. Among the Maori there were believed to be three different immaterial elements of this kind, the *mauri*, the *hau*, and the *ora*, each of which was necessary to well-being and could be affected in different ways, though the relation between them is not clear to us. Natural objects can also have their immaterial essence – their soul-stuff as some writers call it. In Tikopia, when a bundle of green food is laid upon the grave of a dead man, the ancestral spirits are believed to come and to take away the essence of the food, its *ora*, leaving the material substance behind. The people say 'we do not see the spirits do this, but we know that they have taken away the *ora*, because the plants wilt.'

In some societies the vital element is that which is responsible for one's dream adventures, in others the dream counterpart is different again. Dreams often play an important part in African or Oceanic

145

life, not only in building up the theory of the soul and the spirit world, but in guiding action. They are treated as omens, giving warning of the conception of children, their sex, the locality of game sought in hunting, success in undertakings, or sickness and death, and people regulate their conduct accordingly.

Some peoples regard the shadow as a purely physical phenomenon, but others link it up with the human personality, either by giving it special powers of contagion such as the material touch of its owner gives, or by linking it up with the vital principle or even with the soul. The reflection in a mirror or a pool of water can also be an expression of one such immaterial element in personality. The projection of a person into any visual shape, such as a sketch or a photograph, may be disliked by a people because of their belief that such is a projection of an immaterial element of the individual concerned. So, to 'take' a picture of him is interpreted literally as carrying off his personality. Apart from the association with shadow or reflection, one or other of the spirit elements may be located in a definite part of the body, as the stomach, behind the eyes, or in the back. Where the last is the case, hearty back-slapping may have serious consequences!

In almost every human society there appears to be a belief that the individual does not cease to exist at the death of his body, but that he has some continuity in immaterial form. In some societies the ideas of the nature of this continuity of the destination and future of the soul are vague. Life in the next world is not always immortality. The Ila, for instance, believe that a haunting ghost of a dead person can be overcome by a medicine-man, who secures it in a vessel and throws it away on waste land to be consumed by the next grass fire, or into a river to drown. In other societies it is held that the soul lives on and cannot be destroyed. The afterworld may also be well defined, and may comprise a systematic arrangement of zones, lands, or heavens in which the souls of the dead join those of their kinsfolk in particular regions, or those of their social equals in particular ranks or departments. Rarely is there a division according to moral conduct in this world. When there is, it is the morality of the display of wealth and feasting or of bravery in war that takes pride of place, rather than that of goodness in ordinary daily life.

The belief in the persistence of the soul after death has its culmination in the institution of ancestor worship, so common in China and

Polynesia and Africa. Here the spirits of the dead do not simply rest in some Elysium, but take a constant interest in the doings of their descendants, are consulted for their advice on practical problems, and even revisit their people through some human or other medium.

Consider for a moment the beliefs of two peoples in this connection, the Ila of South-East Africa and the Tikopia of Polynesia. The Ila believe in the metamorphosis of men into animals. In accordance with this, men of the lion clan may turn into lions after death, and may leave game that they have killed as a gift to people, or chase old friends for the sport of seeing them run. If the fleeing man stops and addresses the lion by its human name it will turn away and leave him. The Tikopia believe in somewhat similar fashion that the spirit of an ancestor may assume the form of a rat, a bat, a fish, or a bird, and manifest itself to men. A creature that behaves normally is 'just an animal', but when it behaves in a peculiar way, keeping close to a man instead of taking to flight when he tries to scare it, then it is a spirit in this guise, and should be addressed as such. Here is a general belief, that may be termed a dogma, that the spirits of men may take on the form of animals. There are also certain facts needing explanation – that lions do not always refuse to budge from their kill, or injure people whom they chase, or bats and birds do not always fly off when shooed away. They do not behave consistently in their 'natural' way, but sometimes act 'unnaturally'. This unnatural behaviour is reduced to principle by the native belief. The explanation of any particular incident is not itself a matter of dogma, but is an inference from the general principle. In this sense, Tylor was right in stating that animistic beliefs give an explanation of events. In these beliefs in different categories of spirit entities or aspects of the human individual, we can see not merely an intellectual response, as Tylor argued, to two philosophical problems – the nature of dreams and visions, and the difference between life and death. We see rather a complex response to needs of many kinds, to hopes and fears for oneself and for others by whom one's life is made up. Spirit mediumship, metamorphosis, transmigration of souls, reincarnation, are all ways in which the dead are believed to communicate with the living, or to participate again in the life they have left. Through such beliefs people frequently obtain a guide to decisions which they might otherwise find it difficult

147

to take, an escape from ignorance and a feeling of being merely the playthings of chance, and an outlet for emotions.

While it is possible to say how these beliefs work, it is often impossible to say why they should have taken any particular form. The Ila believe in reincarnation; sooner or later almost every person who dies returns to earth in human form, often in that of a grandchild. Ghosts even clamour to be reborn. The precise identity of the new child in terms of its 'real' personality is found by reciting the names of its ancestors when it is held to the breast of its mother. At the moment it begins to suck it is identified as being the returned spirit of the name then mentioned. The Tikopia have no theory of reincarnation. They may name a person after his dead grandfather, or father's brother, or other ancestor, but they do not believe that the living person is then the same as the dead spirit. But they do hold that there can be a particularly close relationship between the living man and the spirit of the dead, who is appealed to by the man to help and protect him in virtue of the name which they bear in common. He and the spirit are spoken of as 'linked names'. In some cases the spirit may manifest himself to men by appearing in the body of his descendant, though he may choose another medium. Like the ghosts of the Ila, those of the Tikopia are believed to be eager to appear in the flesh again, though in the latter case it is not to be reborn, but merely to have the pleasure of eating and drinking, and chewing betel, and of talking. When such a spirit appears it is only for a short time, and he soon takes his leave. It is temporary habitation, not reincarnation. But both Tikopia and Ila beliefs and practices serve to give expression to feelings of affection and interest in kinsfolk who have died, and use these feelings to add colour to the personalities of living individuals and supply them with some sort of standard by which they may act. How the respective beliefs of these two peoples have come into being is beyond our knowledge.

Spiritual beings conceived as non-human in origin are of many kinds. They include spirits of the wild and of the sea; fairies, elves, fauns, water-pixies, goblins, and many other types, in which the individual spirit usually does not receive a personal name, but is regarded as one of a crowd. Then there are spirits of the monster or ogre type, and, again, guardian spirits whose function it is to safeguard the interest of their human wards. In some societies personifi-

148

cations of natural phenomena play a large part in the scheme of religious belief.[3] Some of these spiritual beings are regarded as self-creative, and from their importance in the religious scheme can be given the term of 'gods'. Such a god can be creator, ruler of a spirit world, or, as in much American Indian mythology, a divine trickster.

Each of these types of spiritual beings may correspond to some complex emotional disposition and set of practical problems in the life of the people who believe in them. Wood spirits, fairies, and the like give expression to the fantasy element in human psychology, provide explanation for small pieces of good fortune or mishap, for unaccountable noises heard, for the illusions of fatigue and darkness, and the tendency to see in the movements of Nature analogies with human activity. Stripped of the literary form in which they are so often known nowadays, they must have provided 'reasonable' explanations to a people not highly literary, and to whom the scientific attitude was not so insistently presented as it is to us nowadays. Other types of spirit being are linked with deeper emotions and broader problems. The guardian spirit of the North American Indian, as its name suggests, takes care of a person, instructs him in the way to attain wealth, social eminence, and power, and often appears to him in a vision after prolonged physical privation and searching of the heart. The personifications of natural phenomena are not just the products of a mytho-poetic fancy, but play their part in the attempts of man to control his physical environment for his own economic and social ends. The departmental gods of the Maori were invoked each in his own sphere – the god of the sea for fishing and ocean voyaging, the god of the forests for bird-snaring and canoe-building, the god of agriculture for successful planting and harvests. The creator spirit, again, not only provides intellectual explanation of the origins of the world and of man, but often gives a charter or title to social groups for the particular position that they occupy and the privileges that they exercise. The position of some of these higher gods is not always easy to define, and there has been much controversy about the definition of some of them, and the rôle that they play in native belief. Baiame and Darumulum in Australia, Io in eastern Polynesia, Leza among the Ila and other south-eastern Bantu, Mbori among the Zande, have all been regarded as high gods indicating a recognition by the respective peoples of a power greater than their ordinary pantheon, and an acknowledgment, however dim, of some ultimate moral value in their universe. The position of these deities is not yet entirely clear, particularly because the classification of them as high gods has been championed especially by certain clerics who cannot be regarded as quite free from partisanship. While it is true that no investigator is entirely dispassionate, the researches of some other anthropologists point to the fact that there has been a tendency to invest these deities with attributes more clearcut and more near to our Christian conceptions of the Godhead than are expressed in the beliefs of the peoples themselves. Evans-Pritchard has pointed out that to translate the Zande Mbori as Supreme Being tends to ascribe to him personality, omnipotence, benevolence, and other divine qualities which are by no means clearly formulated by the Zande themselves. When the Zande call upon Mbori it is in situations of fear, anxiety, and despair, but the doctrine about him is vague, and the concept of him overlaps their ideas about ghosts to a large degree.

From all this it would appear that most non-western people at the level of folk belief are essentially polytheistic, and that a true monotheism is not characteristic of them.

Indigenous ideas about their spiritual beings are not merely expressed in the form of doctrinal statements, but are frequently embedded in an elaborate system of mythological tales. These myths are not simply stories preserved for their narrative and dramatic interest. They have a vital function to perform in providing a strongly emotional background to the body of religious belief and to ritual practices. They are an appeal to the past in justification of a great deal of action in the present. The concepts of spiritual beings and their relation to the doings of men involve ideas of supernatural power. These ideas differ from one people to another, but frequently involve beliefs in a quality of sacredness or taboo and in a principle of efficacy of more than a normal human kind. Such is the Oceanic idea of *mana* and the cognate ideas of *wakan* and *orenda* in North America. There has been much discussion of these vernacular terms and their meaning, but it appears as if they represent, not an idea of an all-pervasive abstract power or natural potency so much as the essential characteristic or aspect of activity which consists in the attainment of its end, and its 'working'. I have myself tried to elucidate the meaning of this idea in Polynesia, and could get from Tikopia men explanations of *mana* in terms only such as, 'when we ask the ancestors and gods for the fish to come, or the crops to spring and ripen, and they do so, that is *mana*.' 'When a chief appeals for the wind to fall or the bread-fruit to fruit and it happens, then he is *mana*.' In brief, *mana* is that which is effective or powerful in mystical terms.

Religion cannot be described only in terms of belief. Human faith does not exist in a vacuum, but is applied to ends intended to be successful for human interests. Belief must be translated into rite, faith into action. Marett has said happily, 'savage religion is not so much thought out as danced out' – where dancing may be taken as representative of ritual practice in general. Economic interests, desire for personal distinction, desire to protect oneself and one's associates from illness and misfortune supply the motive forces. As in magic, the rites of religion are a means of bringing belief and desire together by a set procedure. Ritual is the bridge between faith and action.

Of the multitude of religious rites we may mention three – worship of the gods, funeral ritual, and totemic ceremonies.

In our sense worship is apt to mean a bending of the soul towards God in adoration and thanksgiving, in the recognition of His power, His supreme attributes, and His care for us. This somewhat intellec-tual position has tended to obscure the important fact that worship, not only in technologically simple society, has its essentially practical side. It postulates belief in a supernatural being and an attitude in which the superiority of that being to the worshipper is admitted; it uses the appealing forms of prayer and of offering either in propitia-tion or thanksgiving. Sometimes the offering may take the form of a sacrifice of a victim, sometimes merely the bringing of a humble and a contrite heart. But examination of the situation of worship usually reveals some human desire that wants satisfaction, and the offering not infrequently is made in the expectation of a return. The wor-shipper may abase himself before his deity, but in his prayer he uses words of expostulation and command. When he makes his offering it is not only in thanksgiving for past services, but as an indication that these services are expected to continue. The first fruits of the harvest are laid before the god, not only to show that the harvest is appre-ciated, but that other harvests are expected in their turn.

Every society has its funeral rites. When a member of a society dies, a group of people, usually including close kinsfolk of the dead, assem-

151

ble round the corpse, mourn for it, and arrange for its disposal. The assembly is not merely a matter of choice, but is dictated by obligations of a strong sanction. The mourning also is usually not left to the discretion of the mourner's own emotions. He is frequently expected to mourn in prescribed forms, the intensity of his grief is almost codified according to his precise kinship status, and not infrequently he receives some material acknowledgment of these services. It may be thought that the funeral rites would be concerned primarily with the fate of the soul of the dead person, to facilitate his continuity and well-being in the next world. This is often the case, but frequently receives only small attention. There may be little talk about the after-world and of the soul which has departed, and few rites to ensure its safe passage and preservation. Most of the time may be occupied with feasting and exchange of goods, and future arrangements for the members of his family. There is much truth in the view that the essential function of the ritual is to deal with the survivors rather than with the dead. As Radcliffe-Brown has shown for the Andaman Islanders, the death of an individual leaves a gap in the social group and disturbs the emotions of those who still live. The funeral ritual provides a channel for the expression of these emotions, and enforces consideration of the rôle that the individual has played in the social life. In its stress upon the value of an individual to the society of which he is a member the ritual performs one important function, and in assisting the reintegration of the group and recognising the creation of new relationships it performs another.

Totemic ritual is in a different category from the worship of gods and ancestors and from funeral rites. It is much more comprehensive in its nature. In Australia, the field in which it is most elaborate and most deeply welded into the social life of the aboriginal people, totemism is a theory and a practice concerned with the relation between the natural and the social world. It gives a series of principles for the classification of the physical environment, and an organised way of bringing these elements of the environment into a practical relation with man. It provides a theory of origins and a code for utilisation of natural species. It provides also a principle of organisation for the relations of human beings to one another. The ritual associated with the totemic beliefs is complex, and there is great variation in the practices of different tribes. When it takes the form of specific cults two outstanding elements of ritual are often seen. One is the commemoration and recapitulation of the original activities performed by the culture-heroes of the past. These ceremonies, often dramatic and colourful, reproduce the actual incidents of travel, conflict, creation, death, and transformation of men into animals which are believed to have taken place in the dawn of the world. The other, sometimes associated with the first, is the ritual of the *talu*, better known as the *intichiuma*, the name for the ceremony performed in connection with the witchetty grub by the Aranda tribe. These ceremonies are intended to maintain the supply of the totem animal or plant species, and perhaps in some cases to increase it, though the name of 'increase rites' applied to them is not perhaps entirely accurate. Both these types of ritual may be associated with the display of sacred objects frequently ornamented with designs which themselves may be symbolic of the totem or of the doings of the ancestors.

The literature of totemism is vast, from the early statements of McLennan and the great volumes of Sir James Frazer, to the modern analyses of Radcliffe-Brown and Elkin, Stanner and Berndt, and there are many theories of its origin and functions. Sometimes it is classed as a magical phenomenon, sometimes as a religious one. Elements of both appear to be present. Classification apart, it seems clear that on the one hand the totemic ritual gives a system and a stimulus to the aborigine's practical utilisation of his natural surroundings, and on the other, gives occasion for group assembly and the display of social privileges and translates mythology into terms of current practice. On the whole, it symbolises and reaffirms some of the values most fundamental in the economic and social life of the Australian.[4]

This brief sketch of magic and religion has been able only to hint at some of the most important scientific problems they present and their rôle in human life. What has emerged, however, is that they are intimately related to other aspects of human culture, to economics, to technology, to social grouping, to art, and to the primitive equivalent of literature. They bear also on basic human emotions, concerned with the nature of personality and the existence of the individual. What these beliefs and practices which may be termed irrational do is to give a firmness to much rational behaviour, to provide a set of absolutes to which conduct can be referred. In their provision of a sanction for conduct, of a rallying point for man's view of life and the universe, for his relations with his fellows and for his hope for the future, lies much of the explanation for the tenacity with which they are maintained, even when experience would seem to have proved them fallacious.

NOTES

1 Since 1956, the Tikopia have all been Christians, and no longer appeal to their ancestors and traditional gods for economic benefit. For an account of their conversion to Christianity, and its effects upon their traditional rites and beliefs, see my *Rank and Religion in Tikopia*, London, Allen & Unwin, 1970.

2 There is some discrepancy in the usage of the terms 'spirit', 'soul', and 'ghost'. By 'spirit' is sometimes meant all beings or powers, human and non-human in origin; sometimes only those which are non-human. 'Soul' is sometimes used for the spirit of man (and natural objects) before death, with 'ghost' for his spirit after death; sometimes, however, 'soul' is used for his spirit before and after death, and 'ghost' for human spirits which are not at rest and impinge upon human activities.

3 See Plate 18. These eastern Nigerian masked dancers represent several types of spirits. Those with white slender stylised faces, clad in rainbow-type costumes in horizontal bands and patterns of red, yellow, green, black, are female spirits. Though male, the dancers are provided with breasts; their hands are gloved since no part of the body should be exposed. A figure with red and white banded costume and very high carved head-dress is that of a large water-animal spirit. Figures with dress of fibre, shaggy, and with horned or tusked masks, are spirits of bush-cows (buffalo).

4 In a review of the problems of totemism Claude Lévi-Strauss has given a novel theoretical interpretation. Though undervaluing the pragmatic aspect of totemic observances, he has pointed out how totemic classifications can express, or serve as a basis for intellectual categories of other kinds – how totems 'are good to think with' (*Totemism*, trans. Rodney Needham, London, Merlin Press, 1964).

In recent years the traditional hunting and gathering economy of Austra-lian aborigines has been radically curtailed, and so their totemic rituals and beliefs have been much modified.

CHAPTER SEVEN

Anthropology in Modern Life

ANTHROPOLOGY today is not merely the study of the past, or of primitive peoples outside the orbit of civilisation. It has an important rôle to play in the study of spheres of life which westernisation has influenced, and even, perhaps, in the study of our own western institutions, though it has not yet been systematically applied here. In the practical issues of government, education, economic development, and other humanitarian work among peoples all over the world, anthropology is proving that it has a contribution to offer.

Social and Cultural Change

Throughout most of this book we have discussed ways of life as if they were stable, as if institutions continued to function unchanged. This is a convenient assumption, like that of 'other things being equal', of much scientific procedure, to enable us to sort out the effects of particular modes of behaviour. But this does not mean to say that we really think of these institutions as static, that we believe that societies are timeless. Every anthropological investigation is a study at a certain point of time; change is always occurring, whether it be so slow as to be hardly perceptible to ordinary observation, or so rapid as to make it difficult to speak of fixed institutions. Nowadays the study of social and cultural change is an important part of the work of the anthropologist.

The impetus to the processes of change in a society may come from two sources – internal and external. In the internal sphere there are technical inventions, individual struggles for land and power, reformulations of ideas by specially gifted inquiring minds – even a barbaric society may have its philosophers and reformers – pressure of population on the means of subsistence, and perhaps climatic changes. Sometimes the structure of the society does not radically alter in the process. Kinship groups die out and their lands and privileges are inherited according to the recognised principles; new groups are formed by ramification and splitting; privileges are transferred owing to failure to perform the proper obligations, or as the result of unsuccessful rebellion; different families take over tribal leadership. Even customs are dropped out by agreement that they are too burdensome, or on the initiative of a strong-minded chief. Such changes can be noted from the evidence of tribal tradition, and are familiar to every field-anthropologist, who has no reason to doubt their substantial accuracy. Here the 'bony structure' of the society remains unaltered; it is only the flesh and blood that changes. At times, however, the institutional framework does yield, and new organisations for peace or war, or new religious cults arise, leading to a reorientation of the traditional system. Again, when pressure of population, dissatisfaction with existing rule, or love of adventure leads to migration, there may be a readaptation to the new environment, or a change in the political organisation. The many local variations in Polynesian culture are evidence of this. For instance, when the ancestors of the Maori went from Tahiti to New Zealand they had to abandon their bark-cloth for garments of the New Zealand flax, and adopt a different form of tribal organisation with no sovereign chief.

External reasons for change may lie partly within the indigenous field itself, and partly in the expansive power of a neighbouring civilisation. When peoples are in contact with each other they may live side by side at peace, or at war, without their customs being much affected by those of their neighbours. More often they influence one another. They may, like the pastoral Hima and agricultural Iru of Ankole, fit into each other's mode of life while preserving each their own separate institutions. They may, like a Nupe community in northern Nigeria, described by S. F. Nadel, consist originally of distinct cultural groups which, through sharing a common residence, have come to adjust themselves to one another so closely by intermarriage, economic co-operation, and religious interdependence that they now form essentially sections of a single small 'commonwealth'. For this Nadel borrowed a term from biology, and spoke of such a state as 'social symbiosis'. Frequently, when the communities remain separate, they take over ideas about technical processes and ways of behaving from one another, a process that is generally known as diffusion of culture. Some Australian tribes, for instance, have consciously adopted a more complicated system of kinship and marriage groupings from other tribes that have it, apparently because they find it useful to them in social relations with these tribes, and feel some inferiority without it.

More radical, and more important to us today, are the changes wrought by contact of complex civilisations with less advanced peoples. This has often happened in the past, as the influence of Chinese civilisation on the 'barbarians' of its frontiers, of Rome on some of our own ancestors, and of the rule of Islam on the desert tribes of the Near East and of North Africa bear witness. Here it has not been merely a matter of adding new items to a system of which the main fabric still preserves its form, but of revolutionising ways of life and beliefs, and imposing new political and legal institutions. Moreover, these radical changes have often been forced upon people who in the initial stages have been unwilling to accept what has been given to them.

In modern times these cultural compulsives are of great moment. The great technical efficiency of our western civilisation, the desires for extension of sovereignty, for economic exploitation of new natural resources, for new markets for our expanding productive system, and for the religious proselytisation of those whom we conceive to be lacking in certain of the higher values, all have combined to affect, and in some cases to shatter, the framework of institutions and values which other less technically developed people have built up with difficulty over long periods of time.

Anthropology is a young science, barely a century old, and for a time its students were content to examine 'primitive' customs from the point of view of their archaic interest, and to neglect, and even deliberately to rule out of their investigations, the changes that were due to the contact of non-western people with western civilisation. But recently, especially in the last quarter-century, the study of the effects of culture contact, and particularly of the changes produced by these cultural compulsives of modern civilisation, has assumed great energy. Several interests are represented in this: both a scientific and a practical curiosity about the workings of these far-reaching changes, and a hope to be able to formulate laws about them; a belief that in order to control them to the people's best advantage it is

157

necessary to understand them; a belief that in our technical development and our moral values there is much that can be of use to the
more backward peoples. In some cases there is also a relativist standpoint, that the institutions and values of each type of society, even the
simplest, have emerged in response to some particular need, and that,
therefore, they are worthy of being preserved where possible.

The problems of changing cultures are, therefore, being studied
from the point of view of both theoretical and applied anthropology.
On the theoretical side investigation is carried out to establish the
facts and the conditions of change in any community, the factors
responsible for it, the effects on the people's life, and the general
principles which can be used to explain what is happening, and even
predict what will happen. On the applied side there are the questions
about the desirability of these effects, the possibility of producing
some and averting others, or of substituting one set of institutions for
another with least disturbance to the corporate life of the community.

On the theoretical side, the novelty and complexity of the study
are such that although the major problems have been defined, methods
of investigation have been worked out, and much material collected,
the results in the form of general principles have not yet appeared to
any great extent. The material for the study consists mainly of the
observations of anthropologists themselves in the field – what happens, for instance, in a polygynous society [1] when monogamous marriage is made the legal or religious rule; in an agricultural system
when ploughs are introduced to replace the native hoes; in a system
of land tenure when titles to the soil depend upon official registration
and not upon the consensus of tribal opinion or a chief's judgment; in
village and household economy when many of the able-bodied men
go off to work for wages; or in the system of kinship obligations and
mutual economic assistance when new crops are grown for an external market. To supplement this, both local traditions as to what
used to happen in the olden days, and documentary records from
European sources are drawn upon. The interest in the time sequence
of events here brings the anthropologist into the position of an his-
torian, though there is as yet no definite agreement as to how far he
should fulfil this function. By some it is maintained that he should
engage in historical research as far as he can; by others that his main

158

task should be to confine himself to the type of material gained by his personal observation and the verbal information he can obtain. In recent years some historians have been persuaded to apply their special technique to the study of the problems of change in non-western, technically underdeveloped societies. But they are still few, and as yet it seems that the anthropologist should try to fill both rôles.

The results achieved so far in this branch of inquiry have mainly shown the reasons that have led to change in specific institutions, and the effects produced. The theory of the functional interrelation of institutions so strongly stressed by Bronislaw Malinowski has historically been of great importance in such study, but modern analyses focus more on power relationships.[2]

An early instance of the type of result obtained may be cited from the work of Audrey Richards in Zambia. She has shown that among the Bemba the government recognised the chief, but the hereditary religious functionaries who formerly constituted his tribal council were ignored, had no definite status or duties under the new régime, and received no reward for any services that they performed. At a time, then, when a series of new legislative acts were demanded by the government from the chief, he was left without the advice or check of a body which represented tribal opinion. And since many former economic assets of the chief disappeared under the modern conditions, with the abolition of war, and of elephant hunting for ivory, the discouragement of tribute labour, the introduction of some of the European standards of a money economy, the chief could no longer afford to run his advisory and administrative services as before. And the revenues he received from the government were not sufficient to supply this deficiency. The result was that successive governments in Zambia (then Northern Rhodesia) complained that the chiefs failed to make new enactments to better the condition of their people – though it is difficult to see how in the given conditions they could be effectively enforced, despite the fact that the tribal councils still did a great deal of unpaid work.[3]

Another early instance of the disintegrating influence of cultural compulsives from an external source comes from Samoa, in a study by F. M. Keesing. In olden days every Samoan community had as its mistress of ceremonies a high-born virgin known as the *taupo*, who was the pride of the village, and in some degree the centre of its political and social organisation. The *taupo* was given the foremost place of honour in ceremonies, she mixed the kava drink of chiefs and orators on high ritual occasions, she had charge of the entertainment of visitors, she was carefully guarded until marriage and her hand was finally sought by chiefs for her powerful connections as well as her beauty, when the wedding took place with huge exchanges of valued property. The institution of the *taupo* thus served as a means of enhancing social display and hospitality, of intensifying economic life and the distribution of goods, and of securing strategic alliances and valuable kinship connections in the political sphere. Nowadays, however, few *taupo* are to be found, and even in the more conservative communities where one exists, her activities have become much attenuated. The reasons for this show the changes that have come to Samoan life in general, even though the people pride themselves on their conservatism. The missions who were established in Samoa a century ago attacked the *taupo* institutions directly. Her entourage of young women was frowned upon because they were suspected of loose living, and certain of the dances in which she took the most prominent part were prohibited entirely for a time. The method of preparing the kava drink by having the girls of the *taupo*'s entourage chew the root was abandoned in favour of having young men pound it up with stones. The custom of polygyny under which the chiefs took many of the *taupo* as wives was abolished, so that there became 'a glut in the *taupo* marriage market'. Again, the custom of publicly testing the virginity of the *taupo* at her marriage came under the missionary ban. Other indirect factors played an important part. Owing to outlets in Church and other activities the position of women in Samoa has subtly changed, giving them more independence and power in public life. As a result other women, especially those of high rank, have secured privileges that have militated against the pre-eminence of the *taupo* in village life. Then the frequent journeyings from one district to another and one island to another, which gave occasion for elaborate entertainment and exchange of wealth, have tended to be frowned upon by the authorities, and attempts have been made to curb 'wasteful expenditure' that seemed to hamper economic development. Moreover, with the coming of European government and the passing of local warfare, there was no longer the

160

same function for the *taupo* to fulfil in cementing political alliances. The passing of the *taupo* system is not unregretted. A Samoan said, 'It is hard not to be ashamed before visitors if we have no *taupo* to entertain them.'

Such examples give us generalisations of a narrow range, but of suggestive value for comparison. They show how institutions in community life are bound together, so that changes in one may have deep and often unsuspected repercussions upon others. They show also how radically an institution which is well established and vital in the traditional life may break down under the impact of external forces, and yet while there are still traditional needs to be satisfied the people often cling to what remnants of it they can. In this societies appear to differ; some are much more resistant to the processes of change than others are, though we are not yet able to say with assurance in many cases why this should be so.

The interest of anthropologists is not just nostalgic, in survivals of ancient custom, in the institutions of people remote from civilisation and reminiscent of earlier times in the history of man. Most peoples of the world today, even the most underdeveloped, have some kind of active contact with civilisation, especially in its western forms. Many of them try to adapt their society to the economic, political, and social patterns which promise closer relationship with the west in some respects and the possibility of new, more independent rôles in other respects. Sometimes a fairly complete integration is achieved, for individuals, groups, sections, or classes of the population, through their command of wealth, education, or political power. Often there is a specially privileged section who have eminence in all these spheres and who mingle fairly freely with members of the western society. But usually large sections of the people can achieve only inadequate fulfilment of their aims, owing partly to lack of resources and partly to lack of training in the values of the culture they wish to acquire. But there may be also other factors, including their continuing interest in holding on to ways of life with which they are familiar and to which they attach high aesthetic, moral, even spiritual worth. There may be conflict between the values of these ways and those of westernisation. There may be disagreement among the people themselves as to the advisability and possibility of 'assimilation' to the overshadowing alien culture.

161

In any event, social or cultural change cannot be regarded as a mechanical process, nor successful adjustment as a simple matter of introducing 'development', 'enlightenment', and 'progress' to 'backward races'.

For several centuries Christian missionaries have been among the most powerful – and the most publicised – agents of social change. But religious proselytisation is not confined to Christianity. Ever since the days of its founder, Islam has been a religion that seeks converts actively, and in its latest movements it is influencing in a very significant way the culture of the Yoruba, the Mende, and many other West African peoples. Likewise Hinduism, in some respects much more amorphous, and demanding less of its converts, is making great strides among the pagan 'aboriginal' tribes of India.

Apart from religious elements, two powerful sets of forces operate, in the economic and in the political fields, to produce social and cultural changes, in even very isolated communities. One is the set of interests in new, enlarged consumption patterns. The other is the set of interests in new, enlarged control of decisions relating to community affairs. As a result of the first, people alter their habits of production, perhaps quite radically. They go off to work for wages on plantations or in mines. They step up their output of a food commodity such as palm oil or tapioca, and sell the surplus abroad. They engage in the production of an entirely new crop, of no use to them in their domestic economy, such as rubber, copra, or cocoa. With the money they earn they buy a great range of industrially produced goods – cloth, tinned foods, saucepans, cigarettes, electric torches, kerosene lamps, bicycles. They may create new organisational forms to fit the new production schemes – indigenous entrepreneurs of western type with many wage-earners dependent on them; co-operative units for finding and using capital most efficiently; individual land-owners legally secure from the claims of kin and community. On the political side new forms of association may develop, such as village or tribal committees to control local affairs, or representation of nominated or elected type to put the local point of view in a central assembly. Or again, expatriate groups, at work abroad, form associations to promote the welfare of their people at home, partly by the use of 'action group' techniques. In all these, and other ways, new structures are formed in a society, and changes take place in the status system in terms of which people are evaluated. The study of such dynamic aspects of social relations is part of the work of a social anthropologist, and in recent years many analyses of such changes have been made, especially, for example, in Africa, Oceania, and Latin America.

A feature of great importance is the way in which these new structures relate to the traditional, customary social institutions. Sometimes a break is made with the past. After World War II, several communities in New Guinea, such as the Manus of the Admiralty Islands and the Purari of the Papuan Gulf, ostentatiously abolished at one sweep many of their old practices, and even abandoned their traditional villages in order to rebuild their lives anew and emphasise their changed order. More often, elements of the traditional way of life are blended with the new forms. In southern New Guinea the Mailu and some other peoples, having adopted many new forms of association for economic and political purposes, have still kept their old patterns of village alignment, of houses on poles set around a central lane or square, with the clans or other social groups disposed much as in the traditional system. The Melanau of Sarawak, on the other hand, while not deliberately rejecting their old form of domestic life, have dropped their traditional long-house dwelling of apartments set side-by-side in a line under a common roof for scattered individual houses sheltering at most three or four families. This practice was a reaction to an increased demand for sago for export, and a cessation of danger from sudden war raids, which accompanied the establishment of the régime of Raja Brooke. But while the domestic, economic, and (in part) the political system has radically changed over the last half-century, the social forms of kinship and marriage, for example, are still largely of traditional type.

One generalisation of importance which emerges from studies of social and cultural change is that on the whole the people of a community tend to respond most easily to stimuli which have some continuity with, or analogy with, their traditional values and forms of organisation. Even if they are seeking something quite new, they often tend to interpret the resulting organisation in terms of structures and principles with which they are familiar. The Maori of New Zealand, despite the fact that for well over a century they have been acquiring western forms of civilisation, still prefer to conduct many

163

of their public affairs in the style of their forefathers, on the public square, the *marae*, in front of the village meeting-house with its carved boards symbolising tribal ancestors. The occasion may be the funeral of a prominent person, when the old cultural values do receive full recognition. But it may be equally a discussion about building a new sawmill or starting a co-operative dairying enterprise.

The importance of traditional forces is also seen in the way in which after long relationship with an alien culture and apparently radical alteration in their way of life and thought, a people may revert to their ancient practices, or revive elements of such practices and mingle them with modern forms. Examples are the many 'nativistic' movements – practices which in their ritual aspects often combine elements of Christianity or other western institutions with old beliefs and customs in ways that strike the casual observer as travesties of civilised behaviour. Such are the Hauhau cult of the Maori, the Ghost Dance and allied cults of some North American Indian tribes, the Pa Chin Hao of the Chins of Burma, the Watch-Tower movement in its local African form, the 'Cargo cults' and analogous movements in New Guinea and the western Pacific. The genesis and structure of these movements show many differences. But in general they seem to have sprung up largely as a reaction against an apparent lack of control of the situation brought about by western influence. Sometimes they are focused upon a major grievance, such as loss of land; sometimes they appear to have no definite wrong to remedy. Often they have tended to take on a political and anti-European bias. In several, including the Ghost Dance of the Plains Indians and the Hauhau of the Maori, the antagonism led to war. The Mau Mau of the Kikuyu of Kenya, so distressing in its violence and brutality, and conceived in a developed political and military pattern rather than in a ritual one, seems in many respects to belong to the same general category, with its basic land grievance, its oath-taking, its crude, savage symbolism, and the fantastic character of some of its aspirations. Such movements must not be regarded as mere delusion, or as the product of political 'agitation', or as a simple reversion to savagery and atavistic thinking, but as a phenomenon manifesting strain in adaptation. They are attempts at a solution, albeit an ineffective and misjudged one, to the grave difficulties of making old and new institutions, claims, and values meet in a harmonious way. However inarticulate, they are positive reactions of protest, of affirmation of personal dignity, of assertion of knowledge and power. Their emphasis is on the organisation of symbolic as well as practical elements to achieve in some dynamic, dramatic way the hope of the people to control once again their own destiny. Such movements often have much in common with dissident Churches, prophetic and messianic cults, and local religious sects, which also seek a new way out of old troubles, though by primarily ritual means. Moreover, as there can be fundamental disagreement about means, even when ends are common ground, the protagonists of these 'nativistic' and allied movements usually find themselves bitterly opposed by some sections of their own society. Such a struggle, indeed, often canalises and gives expression to ancient status claims and group rivalries characteristic of the traditional society.

About the time that the social anthropologist began to realise the possibilities of his technique for studying social changes in the more technically backward communities, he also came to see its value for studying the more developed rural peoples. Studies have now been made, e.g. of Irish, Welsh, Kurdish, Malay, Indian, and Chinese peasantry; of Bedouin and Arabs; of many of the folk cultures of Latin America and of the West Indies.[4] In them the same kind of problems of kinship, of work, of status, of ritual, are examined as in studies of the more exotic peoples. Emboldened further, some anthropologists have turned from rural to urban investigations, and have examined problems of group structure and values among 'coloured' people in cities of Britain, the United States, and South Africa; of industrial relations and social relations among factory workers; of status and class stratification among white Americans; and even of the culture patterns of Hollywood. The modern social anthropologist in fact can find a laboratory in any social system in which he can apply his intensive techniques of first-hand observation. The study of the institutions of civilisation has already been pursued by a number of sciences – to mention only economics, political science, psychology, and sociology. On the whole these treat of broad phenomena on a large scale. The social anthropologist regards himself usually as allied to the sociologist – though some social scientists disagree about these labels. He may be classed as a sociologist specialising in small-scale first-hand field observation while keeping that holistic framework of ideas about society and culture which he derives from general social theory and his studies of simpler communities. In this form social anthropology might be termed 'micro-sociology', supplementing the 'macro-sociology' of the other sciences. We already know a great deal about the macro-structure of our institutions in western civilisation. What the social anthropologist has to contribute is a more systematic knowledge of their micro-structure and of their organisation – of the precise form of social relationships between people in a factory or a hospital, or a church; and how these relationships actually function in the lives of men and women. Year by year more studies of this kind are being built up into a body of generalisations which, in collaboration with those from the other social sciences, help to throw light on the behaviour of people in our own society.

This bears on the problems of applied anthropology.

Applied Anthropology

Theoretical anthropology, like every other science, has its practical applications. Just as the work of the astronomer can be used for the improvement of navigation, that of the physicist for engineering and radio-telephony, that of the chemist for pharmacy and medicine, so can that of the anthropologist be of use in improving the design of social affairs and remedying difficulties in social relationships. In the earlier days, when social anthropology was concerned mainly with exotic peoples in their relatively undisturbed state, its exponents found little to contribute to aid missionary, trader, or government official in their apparently straightforward task of development. But as unsuspected blocks began to be met in the developmental process, and the peoples concerned began to react in far more complicated ways, often very different from what had been envisaged, a field of application for anthropology was revealed. More and more governments with colonial possessions and other interests in exotic societies, mission bodies, educational institutions, international organisations, and industrial and commercial firms, have been taking advantage of the training which modern anthropology gives, of the publications in anthropology, and of the presence of anthropologists in particular areas, to obtain information of use to them in formulating and carrying out their plans.

From the contact of exotic societies with the west, and from the dynamics of their own internal development, many problems have arisen, calling for the assistance of the social anthropologist. Problems of population control – either of preventing decline, or, in recent years, of providing outlets for growing numbers as an alternative to a policy of family limitation – give scope for elucidation of sex relations and marriage, conception, child-bearing, and child care. Problems of land utilisation involve determination of the complex rights of individuals, groups, chiefs, the community as a whole, even the ancestors; and the way in which kinship structure and inheritance rules may affect the productivity of land. Problems of the effects of industrial employment involve consideration of the labour flow from distant villages, the conditions of women and children left behind (which may include undue agricultural strain on the women and disturbance of authority patterns in regards to children); the new associations formed by labourers in the employment centres, the complex patterns of distribution of their wages. Similar elaborate analysis would be needed in a range of other pressing and difficult matters: problems of the marketing of peasant products; of indebtedness and capital formation; problems of the marriage transaction known as bride-price, and the indigenous use of cattle for non-commercial purposes; problems of witchcraft; of the rise of new prophet cults; and of harmonising school education with local needs.

In these and other problems a knowledge of anthropology can be of use in several ways. In the first place, it helps towards a general understanding of indigenous custom, so that the importance of local attitudes is realised. For example, efforts have been made in the past to abolish the African custom of *lobola*, of giving cattle, goats, or other property in exchange for a wife. Nowadays it has been shown that this custom may help to stabilise a marriage, to give protection to the woman against desertion or ill-treatment, and to establish the legal position of the children. A classic case of the value of an understanding of African belief is given by the Golden Stool of Ashanti. Said to have come down from the sky, the stool was of a kind that Africans ordinarily use, save that it was partially covered with gold. It was cherished as the most sacred possession of the people; it was believed to contain the soul of the Ashanti nation. Though the stool of a chief is normally his throne, the Golden Stool was never sat upon,

167

even by the Asantehene, the King. When its power was evoked the King merely pretended to sit three times on it, and then retired to his own stool, with his arm resting on the Golden Stool. It was never allowed to touch the ground, but was placed on an elephant skin, and covered with a special cloth. On several occasions towards the end of the nineteenth century British officials made attempts to secure the Golden Stool, believing that it was a symbol of supreme authority over the people, to be sat upon as the kingly throne. A governor, indeed, through ignorance, reproached the chiefs that they had not given the Golden Stool to him to sit upon, as the representative of Queen Victoria, instead of his chair. The war that followed owed much to the anger and horror of the Ashanti people at this threatened desecration of their most sacred relic, the symbolic repository of the people's soul.

Twenty years later, after the Stool had been concealed for a long time, it was accidentally dug up by some workmen, with the result that its custodian was persuaded to help in stripping the ornaments from it and selling them. When this was discovered the Ashanti chiefs and people were furious, and demanded the lives of the offenders. Through their government anthropologist, the late Captain Rattray, the government now knew what the Stool really symbolised to the people, and very wisely decided to leave the inquiry and trial in the hands of the Ashanti chiefs themselves. Moreover, though they refused the death penalty, they substituted banishment. And they declared that there was no longer any need to conceal the Stool, since the Ashanti would not now be asked to hand it over.[5]

Understanding promotes tolerance – or should do so – and the knowledge of institutions and beliefs that anthropology has provided has helped in some cases to induce a much less rigid spirit than formerly among those who guide and control the behaviour of others. It has been seen, for instance, that dancing and initiation rites, both usually forbidden in the past, have much that is useful for community life, and that merely to prohibit them may be to disturb the social life deeply. Dr Edwin Smith, a missionary of much experience, and admirably broad-minded, has even suggested that there may sometimes be a case for polygamy. 'The surreptitious concubinage practised by large numbers of professing African Christians is worse than polygamy – it inflicts a greater wrong upon the woman.' He

168

would allow a polygamist who desires to become a Christian to do so without forcing him to discard the women whom he has honourably married, and who are the mothers of his children. And nowadays respect for indigenous values, even though there may not be agreement with them, has gone far. So there must be few Europeans of the temper of the enthusiastic young missionary in the South Seas who blew up a sacred pool with dynamite, and distributed the fish from it, to demonstrate to the recalcitrant and terrified older men that the spirit believed to inhabit it was powerless!

What a knowledge of the principles governing local custom and belief can do in cases where some adjustment must be found between the practices of the people and the values which civilisation brings to the situation, is to suggest substitute ways of behaving instead of immediate and direct prohibition. In New Guinea, for instance, where the taking of a human head was regarded by one tribe as a necessary preliminary to the marriage of a young man, a government anthropologist, by discussion with the older men, was able to get agreement on the substitution of the head of a wild boar instead. To secure this meant initiative and courage on the part of the aspirant to marriage, and satisfied the tribal rule while putting an end to the disruptive acts of head-hunting.

To such earlier instances of applied anthropology in exotic cultures have been added others during and after World War II. Studies of Japanese communities in re-location centres in the United States showed the kinds of strains and resistances that operated in such conditions, and helped to explain why these people were reluctant to work for wages outside the camps, or to be resettled away from their original homes. Studies of Micronesians under American military administration revealed the complexities resulting from the imposition of democratic forms in societies in which leadership still depends largely on hereditary status. Studies among a number of Amerindian communities, such as Hopi, Navaho, Papago, Sioux, under the auspices of the United States Indian Service, have done much to illumine the importance of taking into account traditional patterns and values when programmes of economic and social development are set going. Social anthropologists have been engaged in such socio-economic investigations in many other parts of the world. They have been able to demonstrate the importance of looking at the behaviour

169

of people as part of an intricate social system and not simply as a set of individual responses to the prospects of a more enlightened way of life. It is from this point of view that they have also turned in western society to specialised analyses of human relations in industry and in medicine, paying attention to elements of informal structure which have often been disregarded.

In all these more recent studies the rôle of the anthropologist has usually been less dramatic than in the earlier days. His conclusions on problems, though often of considerable practical use, are usually more in the nature of suggestions than solutions. When the door to development seems stuck he rarely has the key – but he often has found some oil for the hinges. What is meant by this metaphor is that the most useful work of the anthropologist is apt to lie less in coming forward with direct 'answers' to difficult questions of policy and practice, than in making the basic analyses which indicate causes of difficulty and showing how greater conformity to realistic conditions can ease tensions.

A point of some importance arises here. For those who believe in the value of human knowledge as an ultimate good in itself – even though to put it no higher, they base their view on an individual preference of an aesthetic kind – the justification for anthropological science lies in the correctness of the generalisations it produces, in its adequacy to explain some of the complexities of human behaviour. But there are others who argue that the science is to be justified by its practical results, that the anthropologist who is worthy of his hire ought to be helping to find the solutions to difficult problems of administration, or education, or the general improvement of human welfare.

There are difficulties in this view. The conditions in which the problems are set for him are not within the discretion of the anthropologist to vary. He cannot change the broad lines of policy – legal, administrative, economic, religious, educational – even though his researches may lead him to think that they are unsuitable to local needs. He is rather in the position of a doctor asked to advise a patient who says beforehand that, whatever the diagnosis, he must follow a certain type of treatment, and will accept suggestions only on the details of putting it into effect. Again, the final aim of these policies is often undefined. If the anthropologist is asked to help in making a policy of colonial rule more efficient, is this with the ultimate object of fitting the people for self-government, with freedom of choice as to the form of political institutions that they may finally desire, or is it with the aim of simply getting a more cohesive community, with law and order better kept, taxes paid more promptly, and social services more efficiently carried out, all to remain within the framework of an imperial system? When it is argued that anthropology must be ready to give solutions to practical problems, it is too often assumed that the values which the anthropologist should uphold and actively promote are those of our own civilisation. Individualism, technical progress, Christianity, monogamy, are a few of those most generally accepted, and any questioning of them is regarded as subversive of the moral order. Sometimes, though happily less commonly, he is expected also to subscribe to such canons as that of the white man's prestige. But even apart from the last-named attitude, he may regard these general values as not necessarily ideal standards, but simply as ways of complex social behaviour which have emerged in our western civilisation, and have worked well enough here, but which have not been proved to be the most effective institutions or standards for the guidance of other peoples. One has the more need to view with care the moral responsibility that is sometimes thrust upon anthropology, since those who invoke it are often admitted partisans in a struggle of sectional interests – representatives of government, of religious dogma, of economic exploitation, or of local claims. While each has his particular set of assumptions as to where the ultimate reason and good lie, there is a danger that he will be moved to reject as false those generalisations of anthropology which do not happen to serve his special ends. Freedom from the chains of a 'practical' programme is as essential to objective anthropology as it is to other sciences – perhaps even more so than most, since its results can bear so directly upon the lives of men.

This is not to say that anthropological research *may* not be directed to practical ends; it is merely to say that there ought to be no pressure brought to bear that it *should* be so directed. How, then, can the anthropologist be of use in the problems by which we are faced in under-developed countries? His ideal rôle, as I see it, is that of diagnosis and prediction. His function is from the results of his analysis to state what a situation is, and that if certain results are desired, then

171

certain methods should be followed; and alternatively, if certain methods are followed, then certain results will probably occur. But he should not be expected, as a scientist, to agree with the aims that are, in fact, desired. Thus 'value-free', as it were, he is in a stronger position to judge the situation. Of course the term 'value-free' does not mean that the anthropologist himself has no values. But it does mean in this context that he should be recognised as having relative freedom of action in judging what is the right thing to do, by examining and perhaps calling into question ends as well as means. This problem will have a different, though no less important, trend as anthropologists come to be drawn more and more from the body of the peoples under study. Here a risk of loss in immediate objectivity may well be balanced by greater initial familiarity with the problems, and a deeper sense of committal or identification with the ultimate objectives. But the fact that the anthropologist is apt to be identified, as a local person, with given sectional interests, may render his motives more suspect, and put him under more severe pressures, than if he comes from outside the community. There is a strong case, in any event then, for making dispassionate evaluation of situations his aim.

Some modern anthropologists, of radical political convictions, do not agree with such a lack of commitment. But for many others, aquiescence in a radical programme means intellectual hardship, such as sacrifice of critical attitudes towards objectives proclaimed as the official aim of policy. Between such diverse views the argument continues.

Anthropologists do not have a monopoly of tact and understanding in dealing with human affairs, nor can they often provide the desired solution to difficult problems. But at least their grasp of the realities of the structure, organisation, and values of a society does enable anyone who is attempting to change it to ask the right kind of questions and get some answers which will help him to act with discretion. But perhaps the more lasting value of social anthropology as an applied study may be in treating it as a cultural subject for broadening the education of persons of mature mind, enabling them to get a firmer knowledge of the comparative principles of human action. As members of society, we are all interested in attaining as rational a control of our natural and social environment as possible. To this aim anthropology has its contribution to offer, and most of those who are engaged in it see in its discipline something of real value for the understanding and guidance of human affairs.

NOTES

1 Terms for marriage involving varying numbers of spouses have been known since the eighteenth century, and are derived from classical Greek, as follows: *andros*, man, male, husband; *gamos*, mating, marriage; *gyne*, woman, female, wife; *monos*, single; *polos*, much (*polloi*, many). Hence, polyandry, polygyny, monogamy, etc. (*See also* pp. 99, 160).
2 An early set of essays on 'Methods of Study of Culture Contact in Africa', by a group of anthropologists, with a theoretical introduction by Bronislaw Malinowski, was published by the International Institute of African Languages and Cultures, in London, in 1938. A sequence of works indicating how the study of social and cultural change has developed over more than three decades is e.g. the following:
Brown G. & Hutt, B., *Anthropology in Action*, Oxford, 1935
Keesing, F. M., *The South Seas in the Modern World*, New York, 1941
Wilson, G. & Wilson, Monica, *The Analysis of Social Change*, Cambridge, 1945
Spicer, H. (ed.), *Human Problems in Technological Change: A Casebook*, New York, 1952
Mead, Margaret (ed.), *Cultural Patterns and Technical Change*, Tensions and Technology series, UNESCO, Paris, 1953
Gluckman, M., *Custom and Conflict in Africa*, Oxford, Blackwell, 1955
Lloyd, P. C., *Africa in Social Change: Changing Traditional Societies in the Modern World*, Harmondsworth, Penguin, 1967
3 See A. I. Richards, 'Tribal Government in Transition', *Journal Royal African Society*, xxxiv, 1935. Much other material on the Bemba is in Audrey Richards's book *Land, Labour and Diet in Northern Rhodesia*, OUP, 1939.
4 One of the earliest anthropological studies of a western community was Arensburg, C. M. & Kimball, S. T., *Family and Community in Ireland*, Cambridge (Massachusetts), 1940.
5 For a full account of this, see Edwin W. Smith, *The Golden Stool*, 1926.

Bibliography

MUCH important anthropological work is still only available in scientific periodicals, such as *The Journal of the Royal Anthropological Institute* (now *Man*), *American Anthropologist*, *Anthropos*, *Africa, Oceania, Bantu Studies, Journal of the Royal African Society, Journal of the Polynesian Society, Southwestern Journal of Anthropology, Applied Anthropology* (now *Human Organization*), *Ethnology*. Some of the examples in this book have been drawn from articles in these journals.

There are now many books in which general principles of social anthropology are discussed and explained, often from different points of view. The following brief list gives some publications, mainly British, covering major aspects of the subject. Most are recent, but a few of the more useful older works are also included.

Of introductory character are:

Gluckman, Max, *Custom and Conflict in Africa.* Oxford, Blackwell, 1955.

Lienhardt, Godfrey, *Social Anthropology.* Oxford University Press, 1964.

Mair, L. P., *An Introduction to Social Anthropology.* Oxford, Clarendon, 1965.

Beattie, John, *Other Cultures: Aims, Methods and Achievements in Social Anthropology.* London, Cohen & West, 1964; Routledge & Kegan Paul (paper), 1966.

Firth, Raymond, *Elements of Social Organization.* London, Watts, 1951; Tavistock, 1971.

There is a vast literature on race questions. Useful examples of anthropological treatment include:

Little, Kenneth, *Race and Society.* Paris, UNESCO, 1952.

Banton, Michael, *Race Relations.* Social Science Paperbacks, London, Tavistock, 1967.

Banton, Michael, *Racial Minorities.* London, Fontana, 1972.

The history of social anthropology is still to be written. Some preliminary, rather superficial accounts are given by:

Kuper, Adam, *Anthropologists and Anthropology: The British School 1922–1972*. London, Allen Lane, 1973.

Henson, Hilary, *British Social Anthropologists and Language*. Oxford Monographs on Social Anthropology. Oxford, Clarendon, 1974.

A good idea of the scope of social anthropology, with analysis of major problems in the most important fields, is given in the ASA Monographs, published by Tavistock, London, for the Association of Social Anthropologists of the Commonwealth, viz:

Banton, Michael (ed.), no. 1: *The Relevance of Models for Social Anthropology*, 1965; no. 2: *Political Systems and the Distribution of Power*, 1965; no. 3: *Anthropological Approaches to the Study of Religion*, 1966; no. 4: *The Social Anthropology of Complex Societies*, 1966.

Leach, Edmund (ed.), no. 5: *The Structural Study of Myth and Totemism*, 1967.

Firth, Raymond (ed.), no. 6: *Themes in Economic Anthropology*, 1967.

Lewis, I. M. (ed.), no. 7: *History and Social Anthropology*, 1968.

Mayer, Philip (ed.), no. 8: *Socialization: The Approach from Social Anthropology*, 1969.

Douglas, Mary (ed.), no. 9: *Witchcraft Confessions and Accusations*, 1970.

Ardener, Edwin (ed.), no. 10: *Social Anthropology and Language*, 1971.

Needham, Rodney (ed.), no. 11: *Rethinking Kinship and Marriage*, 1971.

Cohen, Abner (ed.), no. 12: *Urban Ethnicity*, 1974.

Other important series in British social anthropology are the London School of Economics Monographs on Social Anthropology, begun in 1940; the Cambridge Papers in Social Anthropology, begun in 1958; and the Oxford Monographs on Social Anthropology, begun in 1963. Some of these are mentioned below.

More technical works:

For those interested in pursuing the subject in depth the following lists represent some of the more important technical publications.

(a) Works on social structure, including kinship and social stratification:

Nadel, S. F., *The Theory of Social Structure*. London, Cohen & West, 1957.

Goody, Jack (ed.), *The Development Cycle in Domestic Groups* (Cambridge Papers in Social Anthropology, no. 1). Cambridge University Press, 1958.

Firth, Raymond, *Social Change in Tikopia*. London, Allen & Unwin, 1959.

Mayer, Adrian C., *Caste and Kinship in Central India*. London, Routledge & Kegan Paul, 1960.

Leach, E. R., *Rethinking Anthropology* (London School of Economics Monographs on Social Anthropology, no. 22). London, Athlone, 1961.

Fortes, Meyer, *Marriage in Tribal Societies* (Cambridge Papers in Social Anthropology, no. 3). Cambridge, University Press, 1962.

Goody, Jack, *Death, Property and the Ancestors*. London, Tavistock, 1962.

Barth, F., *Models of Social Organisation*. London, Royal Anthropological Institute, 1966.

Freedman, Maurice, *Chinese Lineage and Society: Fukien and Kwangtung* (London School of Economics Monographs on Social Anthropology, no. 33). London, Athlone, 1966.

Nakane, Chie, *Kinship and Economic Organization in Rural Japan* (London School of Economics Monographs on Social Anthropology, no. 32). London, Athlone, 1967.

Fox, Robin, *Kinship and Marriage*. Harmondsworth, Penguin, 1967.

Morris, H. S., *The Indians in Uganda: Caste and Sect in a Plural Society*. London, Weidenfeld & Nicolson, 1968.

Gellner, Ernest, *Saints of the Atlas*. London, Weidenfeld & Nicolson, 1969.

Nukunya, G. K., *Kinship and Marriage among the Anlo Ewe* (London School of Economics Monographs on Social Anthropology, no. 37). London, Athlone, 1969.

Leach, E. R., *Political Systems of Highland Burma* (London School of Economics Monographs on Social Anthropology, no. 44) (paper). London, Athlone, 1970. (First pub. London, Bell, 1954.)

Dumont, Louis, *Homo Hierarchicus: The Caste System and its Implications*. London, Weidenfeld & Nicolson, 1970.

Fortes, Meyer, *Kinship and the Social Order*. London, Routledge & Kegan Paul, 1970.

Barnes, J. A., *Three Styles in the Study of Kinship*. London, Tavistock, 1971.

Bloch, Maurice, *Placing the Dead: Tombs, Ancestral Villages and Kinship Organization in Madagascar*. London, Seminar Press, 1971.

Philpott, Stuart B., *West Indian Migration: The Montserrat Case* (London School of Economics Monographs on Social Anthropology, no. 47). London, Athlone, 1973.

(b) Anthropological studies in the European and Mediterranean field:

Pitt-Rivers, J. A., *The People of the Sierra/Spain/*. London, Weidenfeld & Nicolson, 1954.

Frankenberg, Ronald, *Village on the Border: A Social Study of Religion, Politics and Football in a North Wales Community*. London, Cohen & West, 1957.

Stirling, Paul, *Turkish Village*. London, Weidenfeld & Nicolson, 1965.

Firth, Raymond; Hubert, Jane; Forge, Anthony, *Families and Their Relatives: Kinship in a Middle-Class Sector of London*. London, Routledge & Kegan Paul, 1969.

Davis, J., *Land and Family in Pisticci/Italy/* (London School of Economics Monographs on Social Anthropology, no. 48). London, Athlone, 1973.

(c) Studies in economic anthropology:

Belshaw, Cyril S., *Traditional Exchange and Modern Markets*. Englewood Cliffs, N.J., Prentice-Hall, 1965.

Swift, M. G., *Malay Peasant Society in Jelebu* (London School of Economics Monographs on Social Anthropology, no. 29). London, Athlone, 1965.

Firth, Raymond, *Malay Fishermen: Their Peasant Economy*. London, Routledge & Kegan Paul (rev. ed.), 1966.

Firth, Rosemary, *Housekeeping Among Malay Peasants* (London School of Economics Monographs on Social Anthropology, no. 7) (rev. ed.). London, Athlone, 1966.

Wallman, Sandra, *Take Out Hunger: Two Case Studies of Rural Development in Basutoland* (London School of Economics Monographs on Social Anthropology, no. 39). London, Athlone, 1969.

Ortiz, Sutti R., *Uncertainties in Peasant Farming: A Colombian Case* (London School of Economics Monographs on Social Anthropology, no. 46). London, Athlone, 1973.

Sahlins, Marshall, *Stone Age Economics*. London, Tavistock, 1974.

(d) Studies in political anthropology:

Schapera, I., *Government and Politics in Tribal Societies*. London, Watts, 1956.

Smith, M. G., *Government in Zazzau*. London, Oxford University Press, 1960.

Gluckman, M., *Politics, Law and Ritual in Tribal Societies*. Oxford, Blackwell, 1965.

Bailey, F. G., *Stratagems and Spoils: A Social Anthropology of Politics*. Oxford, Blackwell, 1969.

Fallers, Lloyd A., *Law Without Precedent: Legal Ideas in Action in the Courts of Colonial Busoga*. Chicago University Press, 1969.

Balandier, Georges, *Political Anthropology* (trans. A. M. Sheridan Smith from Fr. ed. of 1967). Harmondsworth, Penguin, 1972.

Cohen, Abner, *Two-Dimensional Man: An Essay on the Anthropology of Power and Symbolism in Complex Society*. London, Routledge & Kegan Paul, 1974.

(e) Studies in thought and religion:

The field of mystical thought and symbolism concerned especially with myth, religion and ritual is very complex, and has been the object of many anthropological studies. Among those of special interest, including a couple of early classics, are:

Evans-Pritchard, E. E., *Witchcraft, Oracles and Magic among the Azande*. Oxford, Clarendon, 1937.

Forde, Daryll (ed.), *African Worlds: Studies in the Cosmological Ideas and Social Values of African People*. International African Institute. London, Oxford University Press, 1954.

Lienhardt, Godfrey, *Divinity and Experience: The Religion of the Dinka*. Oxford, Clarendon, 1961.

Fortes, M. & Dieterlen, G., *African Systems of Thought*. International African Institute. London, Oxford University Press, 1965.

Douglas, Mary, *Purity and Danger*. London, Routledge & Kegan Paul, 1966.

Leach, E. R. (ed.), *Dialectic in Practical Religion* (Cambridge Papers in Social Anthropology, no. 5). Cambridge University Press, 1968.

Leach, E. R., *Genesis as Myth and Other Essays*. London, Cape, 1969.

Burridge, Kenelm, *New Heaven New Earth: A Study of Millenarian Activities*. Oxford, Blackwell, 1969.

Turner, Victor W., *The Ritual Process: Structure and Anti-Structure*. Chicago, Aldine, 1969.

Firth, Raymond, *Rank and Religion in Tikopia: A Study in Polynesian Paganism and Conversion to Christianity*. London, Allen & Unwin, 1970.

Lewis, I. M., *Ecstatic Religion: An Anthropological Study of Spirit Possession and Shamanism*. Harmondsworth, Penguin, 1971.

Needham, Rodney, *Belief, Language and Experience*. Oxford, Blackwell, 1972.

Firth, Raymond, *Symbols, Public and Private*. London, Allen & Unwin, 1973.

La Fontaine, J. (ed.), *The Interpretation of Ritual: Essays in Honour of A. I. Richards*. London, Tavistock, 1973.

Index

181